# Overcoming Thyroid Cancer

A comprehensive guide to living in wellness

**Dr. Daniel Thompson**

Copyright

# TABLE OF CONTENT

# Introduction

"In the intricate tapestry of human health, the tale of thyroid cancer unfolds as a story of resilience, medical advancements, and the indomitable spirit of those navigating the intricate pathways of their bodies. This book delves into the nuanced landscape of thyroid cancer, weaving together the threads of scientific understanding, personal narratives, and the relentless pursuit of innovative treatments.

As we embark on this exploration, we journey through the delicate butterfly-shaped gland that is the thyroid—a seemingly small yet profoundly influential organ nestled in the neck. Thyroid cancer, a formidable adversary, disrupts the harmony of this vital endocrine system, demanding attention, understanding, and a collective effort to confront its complexities.

Within these pages, readers will discover the intricacies of thyroid cancer—from its subtle whispers to the courageous stories of individuals facing the diagnosis head-on. We unravel the science behind the disease, exploring diagnostic breakthroughs, treatment modalities, and the ongoing pursuit of a deeper comprehension of thyroid cancer's multifaceted nature.

This book is not merely a collection of facts; it is an empathetic journey into the lives touched by thyroid cancer, a beacon of knowledge for those seeking to understand, cope, and triumph in the face of this formidable adversary. Together, let us illuminate the shadows of thyroid cancer, fostering awareness, compassion, and a shared commitment to conquering this chapter in the vast narrative of human health."

## Overview of Thyroid Cancer

Thyroid cancer, a condition arising from the abnormal growth of cells in the thyroid gland, represents a diverse spectrum of malignancies with distinctive characteristics. Nestled in the neck, the butterfly-shaped thyroid plays a pivotal role in regulating metabolism and hormone production. Thyroid cancer often begins imperceptibly, with subtle symptoms or the discovery of nodules during routine examinations.

Comprising various subtypes, including papillary, follicular, medullary, and anaplastic, each presents unique challenges in diagnosis and treatment. Papillary thyroid cancer, the most prevalent form, generally carries a favorable prognosis, while follicular and medullary types introduce complexities in their behavior and management.

Diagnosis involves imaging studies, biopsies, and molecular testing to discern the cancer's specific features. Treatment modalities range from surgery and radioactive iodine therapy to targeted medications, each tailored to the cancer's characteristics and the patient's overall health.

Amidst the medical landscape, patient narratives intertwine with scientific advancements, illustrating the emotional and physical dimensions of thyroid cancer. Ongoing research endeavors seek to unravel the intricacies of this disease, fostering hope for improved detection, personalized therapies, and enhanced outcomes. This overview encapsulates the dynamic nature of thyroid cancer, urging collective awareness and understanding to illuminate the path toward effective management and, ultimately, a triumph over this intricate challenge.

## Importance of Early Detection

Early detection of thyroid cancer holds paramount significance in improving patient outcomes and reducing the impact of the disease. Detecting thyroid cancer in its initial stages often allows for more effective treatment and increases the likelihood of successful outcomes.

1. Treatment Efficacy: Identifying thyroid cancer early provides an opportunity for less invasive and more targeted treatment options. Surgical interventions, such as thyroidectomy, may be more successful when the cancer is confined to the thyroid gland.

2. Reduced Complications: Early detection minimizes the risk of complications associated with advanced stages of thyroid cancer. Timely intervention can prevent the spread of cancer to surrounding tissues and lymph nodes.

3. Improved Prognosis: The prognosis for thyroid cancer is generally favorable, especially when diagnosed early. Early-stage thyroid cancers, particularly papillary and follicular types, often respond well to treatment, leading to a higher chance of long-term survival.

4. Quality of Life: Early detection and treatment contribute to a better quality of life for individuals with thyroid cancer. It can reduce the need for extensive treatments and decrease the emotional and physical burden on patients.

5. Prevention of Spread: Identifying and treating thyroid cancer in its early stages helps prevent the spread of cancer cells to distant organs, which is crucial for managing the disease effectively.

Regular screenings, self-examinations, and prompt medical attention for symptoms such as thyroid nodules or changes in the neck are essential components of early detection efforts. Ultimately, early detection not only saves lives but also enhances the overall well-being of individuals diagnosed with thyroid cancer.

# Chapter 1

# Understanding Thyroid Cancer

Chapter 1, "Understanding Thyroid Cancer," delves into the intricate landscape of this disease, unraveling the complexities of the thyroid gland and the diverse spectrum of thyroid cancers. Exploring the genesis of these malignancies and the factors influencing their development, the chapter navi nogates through early symptoms, diagnostic approaches, and the significance of molecular testing. Readers embark on a journey of comprehension, laying the foundation for the nuanced discussions on treatment modalities, patient perspectives, and ongoing research. As we navigate the terrain of understanding thyroid cancer, a deeper awareness unfolds, fostering empathy, knowledge, and a foundation for the chapters that follow.

## Types of Thyroid Cancer

Thyroid cancer manifests in several distinct types, each characterized by its unique features, behaviors, and implications for diagnosis and treatment.

1. Papillary Thyroid Cancer (PTC): The most common type, PTC arises from follicular cells and generally exhibits slow growth. It often presents as thyroid nodules and has a favorable prognosis with high survival rates.

2. Follicular Thyroid Cancer (FTC): Arising from follicular cells, FTC tends to spread to blood vessels. While it has a good prognosis for localized cases, distant metastasis can pose challenges.

3. Medullary Thyroid Cancer (MTC): Originating in the C cells that produce calcitonin, MTC is less common. It can be associated with genetic syndromes and requires specialized treatment.

4. Anaplastic Thyroid Cancer (ATC): Highly aggressive and rare, ATC often grows rapidly and has a poor prognosis. Treatment may involve a

combination of surgery, radiation, and chemotherapy.

5. Thyroid Lymphoma: A rare form of thyroid cancer originating in immune system cells within the thyroid. It necessitates unique treatment approaches, including chemotherapy and immunotherapy.

6. Thyroid Hürthle Cell Carcinoma: A subtype of follicular thyroid cancer with distinct Hürthle cells. It can behave more aggressively than typical FTC.

Understanding these varied types is pivotal for accurate diagnosis and tailored treatment plans. Diagnostic tools, including fine-needle aspiration (FNA) biopsies and molecular testing, help discern the specific type, guiding healthcare professionals in providing the most effective interventions. As research advances, ongoing efforts strive to uncover the molecular intricacies of each subtype, paving the way for more targeted therapies and improved outcomes for individuals facing the diverse challenges of thyroid cancer

Causes and Risk Factors

The causes and risk factors of thyroid cancer are multifaceted, influenced by a combination of genetic, environmental, and lifestyle elements.

1. Genetic Factors: Inherited genetic mutations play a role in some cases, particularly with medullary thyroid cancer (MTC) and familial forms of differentiated thyroid cancers. The presence of certain genetic syndromes, such as Multiple Endocrine Neoplasia (MEN), increases the risk.

2. Radiation Exposure: Exposure to ionizing radiation, especially during childhood, is a well-established risk factor. This can be from medical treatments (such as radiation therapy for head and neck cancers) or environmental sources.

3. Gender and Age: Thyroid cancer occurs more frequently in women than men. The risk also tends to increase with age, with most cases diagnosed in people between 25 and 65 years old.

4. Thyroid Conditions: Certain thyroid conditions, such as goiter (enlarged thyroid) and chronic inflammation (thyroiditis), may elevate the risk. This is particularly true for differentiated thyroid cancers like papillary and follicular types.

5. Iodine Deficiency or Excess: Both insufficient and excess iodine intake have been associated with an increased risk of thyroid cancer. Iodine is crucial for thyroid function, and imbalances can impact thyroid health.

6. Family History: A family history of thyroid cancer may elevate the risk, suggesting a genetic predisposition. However, most cases occur sporadically without a familial link.

7. Hormonal Factors: Hormonal influences, such as estrogen levels, might contribute to the higher incidence of thyroid cancer in women. Pregnancy and the use of hormonal therapies could play a role.

8. Dietary Factors: While the link is not fully understood, some studies suggest dietary factors, including low selenium intake and high consumption of certain foods, may influence thyroid cancer risk.

9. Obesity: There is evidence that obesity may be associated with an increased risk of thyroid cancer, particularly more aggressive forms.

Understanding these causes and risk factors is crucial for preventive strategies, early detection, and personalized approaches to managing thyroid cancer risk. Regular medical check-ups, awareness of familial history, and minimizing exposure to known risk factors are essential components of thyroid cancer prevention.

## Signs and Symptoms

Thyroid cancer is a relatively rare form of cancer that originates in the cells of the thyroid gland, a butterfly-shaped organ located at the base of the neck. Understanding the signs and symptoms associated with thyroid cancer is crucial for early detection and effective management.

One of the primary manifestations of thyroid cancer is the presence of a palpable lump or swelling in the neck. This lump, often referred to as a thyroid nodule, may be noticeable during self-examination or discovered by a healthcare professional. While not all thyroid nodules are cancerous, it is essential to investigate any unusual growth to determine its nature and potential threat.

Alterations in voice can also serve as a symptom of thyroid cancer. The vocal cords are in close proximity to the thyroid gland, and the growth of cancerous cells can impact their function. Individuals with thyroid cancer may experience hoarseness or changes in their voice quality, prompting further medical evaluation.

Difficulty swallowing, or dysphagia, is another symptom associated with thyroid cancer. As the tumor grows, it may impede the normal swallowing process, causing discomfort or a sensation of a lump in the throat. Persistent difficulty in swallowing should be promptly addressed to rule out thyroid cancer or other underlying issues.

Neck pain, though less common, can be a symptom of advanced thyroid cancer. As the tumor progresses, it may invade surrounding tissues and nerves, leading to discomfort or pain in the neck region. However, it's crucial to note that neck pain is a less specific symptom and can be attributed to various conditions.

Thyroid cancer can also present with changes in thyroid function, although this is not always the case. Some individuals may experience hyperthyroidism, characterized by increased production of thyroid hormones, while others may develop hypothyroidism, marked by insufficient hormone production.

Regular medical check-ups and thorough examination of any concerning symptoms are essential for the early detection of thyroid cancer. Diagnostic procedures, including imaging studies, biopsies, and blood tests, play a pivotal role in confirming the presence of cancer and determining its specific type and stage.

In summary, thyroid cancer manifests through a variety of signs and symptoms, ranging from palpable nodules and voice changes to difficulty swallowing and, in advanced cases, neck pain. Timely medical attention and diagnostic evaluation are crucial for accurate diagnosis and effective management of thyroid cancer.

# Diagnosis and Staging

## Diagnostic Tests

Diagnostic tests for thyroid cancer include:

1. Physical Examination:
   Healthcare professionals may conduct a thorough examination of the neck to detect any palpable lumps or abnormalities in the thyroid gland.

2. Thyroid Ultrasound:
   An ultrasound scan provides detailed images of the thyroid gland, helping to identify the size, shape, and characteristics of any nodules. This imaging technique assists in distinguishing between benign and malignant nodules.

3. Fine Needle Aspiration (FNA) Biopsy:
   FNA involves using a thin needle to extract a small tissue sample from a thyroid nodule. The sample is then examined under a microscope to determine if cancerous cells are present.

4. Blood Tests:
  Blood tests, such as thyroid function tests, measure levels of thyroid hormones and thyroid-stimulating hormone (TSH). While not a definitive cancer diagnosis, abnormal hormone levels may suggest thyroid dysfunction, prompting further investigation.

5. Thyroid Scan:
  A thyroid scan involves the administration of a small amount of radioactive iodine, which is taken up by thyroid cells. Abnormalities in the uptake pattern may indicate the presence of cancerous cells.

6. CT Scan or MRI:
  These imaging studies help assess the extent of thyroid cancer and whether it has spread to surrounding tissues or lymph nodes.

7. Genetic Testing:
  In some cases, genetic testing may be recommended to identify specific genetic mutations associated with an increased risk of thyroid cancer.

8. Laryngoscopy:

If voice changes are a concern, a laryngoscopy may be performed to examine the vocal cords and assess any potential impact from the thyroid tumor.

9. PET Scan:
   Positron emission tomography (PET) scans can be used to detect distant metastases by highlighting areas with increased metabolic activity.

These diagnostic tests, often used in combination, play a crucial role in confirming the presence of thyroid cancer, determining its type and stage, and guiding appropriate treatment strategies. It's important for individuals with suspected thyroid cancer to consult with healthcare professionals who can tailor the diagnostic approach to their specific case.

## Stages of Thyroid Cancer

Thyroid cancer is staged based on the extent of tumor growth and whether it has spread to other parts of the body. The most commonly used staging system is the TNM system, which considers the size of the primary tumor (T), the involvement of nearby lymph nodes (N), and the presence of distant metastasis (M). The stages are typically numbered from I to IV, with higher numbers indicating more advanced disease.

1. Stage I:
   - T1: The tumor is limited to the thyroid and is 2 cm or smaller.
   - N0: No regional lymph node involvement.
   - M0: No distant metastasis.

2. Stage II:
   - T2: The tumor is larger than 2 cm but not larger than 4 cm and is still confined to the thyroid.
   - N0: No regional lymph node involvement.
   - M0: No distant metastasis.

3. Stage III:
   - T3: The tumor is larger than 4 cm or extends beyond the thyroid gland.
   - N0 or N1a: No regional lymph node involvement or involvement limited to pretracheal, paratracheal, or prelacy geal/delphian lymph nodes.
   - M0: No distant metastasis.

4. Stage IVA:

- T4a: The tumor extends beyond the thyroid gland and invades nearby structures, such as the trachea, esophagus, or larynx.
- N0 or N1a: No regional lymph node involvement or involvement limited to pretracheal, paratracheal, or prelaryngeal/delphian lymph nodes.
- M0: No distant metastasis.

5. Stage IVB:
- Any T: The tumor may be any size and may have invaded nearby structures.
- N1b: Lymph node involvement in lateral neck compartments.
- M0: No distant metastasis.

6. Stage IVC:
- Any T: The tumor may be any size and may have invaded nearby structures.
- Any N: Lymph node involvement in any neck compartment.
- M1: Distant metastasis is present.

Staging helps guide treatment decisions and provides prognostic information. Early-stage thyroid cancer (Stages I and II) often has a favorable prognosis, while advanced stages (III and IV) may require more aggressive treatments. It's important for individuals diagnosed with thyroid cancer to discuss their specific stage and treatment options with their healthcare team

# Chapter 2

# Conventional Treatment Options

This chapter illuminates the core strategies in the battle against thyroid cancer, exploring a spectrum of conventional treatments. From precision surgeries such as thyroidectomy to the targeted potency of radioactive iodine therapy, readers embark on a journey through established modalities. We delve into the pivotal role of hormone replacement post-surgery, the strategic use of external beam radiation, and the evolving landscape of chemotherapy. Moreover, the chapter unravels the promise held by targeted therapies and sheds light on the dynamic realm of clinical trials. Navigating through these conventional avenues, readers gain a comprehensive understanding to inform their choices and empower their journey against thyroid cancer.

# Surgery

Thyroid cancer surgery, known as thyroidectomy, is a critical component of the comprehensive treatment approach for individuals diagnosed with thyroid cancer. The thyroid, a butterfly-shaped gland located in the neck, plays a crucial role in regulating metabolism through hormone production. When cancer affects the thyroid, surgical intervention is often necessary.

1. **Types of Thyroidectomy**:
   - Total Thyroidectomy: Removal of the entire thyroid gland is common, especially for larger tumors or cases where cancer has spread beyond the thyroid.
   - Partial Thyroidectomy (Hemithyroidectomy): Removal of one lobe of the thyroid gland may be sufficient for smaller tumors confined to one side.

2. **Lymph Node Dissection:**
   - In cases where cancer has spread to nearby lymph nodes, a neck dissection may be performed to remove affected nodes.
   - Central compartment dissection focuses on nodes around the thyroid, while lateral compartment dissection involves nodes further away.

### 3. Minimally Invasive Techniques:
   - Endoscopic or robotic-assisted thyroidectomy aims to reduce scarring and recovery time compared to traditional open surgery.
   - These techniques involve small incisions and specialized instruments controlled by the surgeon.

### 4. Postoperative Considerations:
   - Hormone Replacement Therapy (HRT): Total thyroidectomy necessitates lifelong thyroid hormone replacement to maintain metabolic balance.
   - Calcium Monitoring: The surgery may impact the parathyroid glands, leading to calcium level changes. Monitoring and supplementation may be required.

### 5. Complications and Risks:
   - Possible complications include damage to vocal cords or parathyroid glands, bleeding, infection, or scarring.
   - Thorough preoperative assessments and skilled surgical techniques aim to minimize these risks.

### 6. Recovery and Follow-up:
   - Recovery times vary but generally involve a hospital stay and a period of restricted activities.

- Regular follow-up appointments and monitoring are crucial to track thyroid hormone levels, detect potential recurrence, and manage any postoperative issues.

## 7. Multidisciplinary Approach:
- Collaboration among endocrinologists, surgeons, oncologists, and other specialists ensures a comprehensive and tailored treatment plan.

## 8. Emotional and Psychological Impact:
- Thyroid cancer diagnosis and treatment can have emotional and psychological effects. Support groups and counseling may be beneficial.

## Radiation Therapy

Radiation therapy is a crucial component in the treatment of various cancers, including thyroid cancer. Here's an overview:

## 1. Purpose:
- Radiation therapy, also known as radiotherapy, uses high doses of radiation to target and destroy cancer cells.

- In thyroid cancer, it is commonly employed after surgery to eliminate any remaining cancer cells and reduce the risk of recurrence.

## 2. Types of Radiation Therapy:
- External Beam Radiation: A focused beam of radiation is directed at the tumor from outside the body. Precise targeting helps minimize damage to surrounding healthy tissues.
- Internal Radiation (Brachytherapy): Radioactive material is placed directly inside or very close to the tumor. This method is less common in thyroid cancer.

## 3. Indications for Radiation Therapy in Thyroid Cancer:
- High-Risk Cases: Patients with aggressive or advanced forms of thyroid cancer may receive radiation to prevent recurrence.
- Incomplete Surgical Removal: If the entire tumor couldn't be removed during surgery, radiation can target remaining cancer cells.

## 4. Procedure and Sessions:
- Patients usually undergo a simulation session to precisely plan the treatment, including positioning and targeting.

- Daily sessions, spanning several weeks, deliver controlled doses of radiation. Treatment frequency and duration depend on the type and stage of cancer.

## 5. Side Effects:
- Short-Term Effects: Fatigue, skin irritation, and difficulty swallowing are common, often resolving after treatment completion.
- Long-Term Effects: Potential for damage to nearby tissues, including the salivary glands and thyroid gland remnants.

## 6. Combination with Other Treatments:
- Radiation therapy is often combined with surgery and may precede or follow chemotherapy, depending on the specific characteristics of the cancer.

## 7. Monitoring and Follow-up:
- Regular follow-up appointments and imaging tests help monitor the response to radiation therapy and detect any signs of recurrence.

## 8. Advancements in Radiation Oncology:
- Technological advances, such as intensity-modulated radiation therapy (IMRT) and proton

therapy, enhance precision and reduce collateral damage to healthy tissues.

## 9. Patient Support:
   - Radiation therapy can be emotionally and physically taxing. Supportive care, including counseling and symptom management, is essential for the well-being of patients.

## Chemotherapy

Chemotherapy is a systemic treatment involving the use of drugs to destroy or slow the growth of cancer cells throughout the body. Here are key points to consider:

## 1. Purpose:
   - Chemotherapy is often employed in thyroid cancer when cancer cells have spread beyond the

thyroid gland or if other treatments haven't been fully effective.
   - It aims to target rapidly dividing cells, including cancer cells, to inhibit their growth.

2. Administration:
   - Medications can be administered orally, intravenously, or through injections, allowing them to circulate in the bloodstream and reach cancer cells throughout the body.

3. Indications for Thyroid Cancer:
   - Chemotherapy is typically reserved for aggressive or advanced forms of thyroid cancer that do not respond well to surgery or radiation.
   - Anaplastic thyroid cancer, in particular, may be treated with chemotherapy due to its rapid growth.

4. Combination Therapy:
   - Often used in combination with surgery and/or radiation therapy to address different aspects of cancer treatment.
   - The specific drugs chosen depend on the type and stage of thyroid cancer.

5. Side Effects:

- Common Side Effects: Nausea, fatigue, hair loss, and immune suppression are common side effects. These are often temporary and can be managed with supportive care.
- Long-Term Effects: Potential for infertility, nerve damage, or increased risk of other cancers in some cases.

6. Duration and Cycles:
- Chemotherapy is typically delivered in cycles, allowing the body time to recover between treatments.
- The overall duration of treatment varies based on the individual's response and the specific cancer characteristics.

7. Monitoring and Adjustments:
- Regular monitoring through blood tests and imaging helps assess the effectiveness of chemotherapy.
- Adjustments to the treatment plan may be made based on the patient's response and any observed side effects.

8. Advancements in Chemotherapy:
- Ongoing research leads to the development of targeted therapies and immunotherapies, which aim

to be more selective in attacking cancer cells while minimizing damage to healthy cells.

9. Emotional Impact:
   - Coping with the emotional and psychological impact of chemotherapy is a significant aspect of cancer treatment. Support groups and counseling play a crucial role in addressing these challenges.

# Chapter 3

# Innovative Treatment Approaches

In this chapter, we embark on a journey into the frontier of thyroid cancer treatment, where innovation takes center stage. Departing from conventional approaches, we explore cutting-edge and unconventional therapies that have emerged as beacons of hope in the fight against thyroid cancer. From nanotechnology and genetic interventions to novel uses of light and sound, these groundbreaking treatments promise to redefine the landscape of thyroid cancer care. Join us as we delve into the realms of innovation, pushing the boundaries of what is possible and offering new rays of optimism for patients and practitioners alike.

## Targeted Therapies

Targeted therapies for thyroid cancer represent a more focused and precise approach in treating specific molecular and genetic abnormalities associated with cancer. Here's an overview:

1. Molecular Targets:
   - Targeted therapies focus on specific molecules involved in the growth and survival of cancer cells.
   - In thyroid cancer, common molecular targets include mutated genes like BRAF and RET.

2. BRAF Inhibitors:
   - BRAF mutations are prevalent in papillary thyroid cancer.
   - Drugs like vemurafenib and dabrafenib inhibit the activity of mutated BRAF, hindering cancer cell growth.

3. RET Inhibitors:
   - RET gene alterations are found in medullary thyroid cancer.
   - Drugs like vandetanib and cabozantinib target the abnormal RET signaling pathway, impeding cancer progression.

4. Tyrosine Kinase Inhibitors (TKIs):
   - TKIs, such as sorafenib and lenvatinib, block signals within cancer cells and the surrounding blood vessels, inhibiting tumor growth.

- These are often used in advanced cases of differentiated thyroid cancer.

5. Immunotherapies:
   - Immune checkpoint inhibitors like pembrolizumab and nivolumab, though not thyroid cancer-specific, have shown promise in certain cases, particularly in poorly differentiated or anaplastic thyroid cancers.

6. Combination Therapies:
   - Some patients may receive a combination of targeted therapies or a combination of targeted therapy with traditional treatments like surgery or radiation.

7. Response Monitoring:
   - Regular monitoring, including imaging studies and molecular testing, helps assess the response to targeted therapies.
   - Adjustments to the treatment plan may be made based on the evolving nature of the cancer.

8. Side Effects:
   - Targeted therapies often have different side effect profiles compared to traditional chemotherapy, but they can still cause adverse

effects such as hypertension, skin problems, and fatigue.

9. Precision Medicine:
   - The advent of precision medicine allows for tailored treatments based on the specific genetic makeup of an individual's cancer.
   - Molecular testing helps identify potential targets, guiding the choice of targeted therapies.

10. Research and Future Directions:
   - Ongoing research explores additional molecular targets and novel therapeutic approaches for thyroid cancer.
   - Clinical trials play a crucial role in evaluating the efficacy and safety of emerging targeted therapies.

Immunotherapy

Immunotherapy is an innovative approach in the realm of cancer treatment, and its application to thyroid cancer is a subject of increasing interest. Thyroid cancer, though often treatable with surgery, radioactive iodine therapy, and hormone therapy, may not respond well to traditional treatments in some cases. This is where immunotherapy comes into play.

One of the key principles behind immunotherapy is leveraging the body's own immune system to recognize and attack cancer cells. In the context of thyroid cancer, researchers are exploring various immunotherapeutic strategies. One notable avenue is immune checkpoint inhibitors. These drugs target specific proteins on immune cells and cancer cells, essentially "releasing the brakes" on the immune system, allowing it to more effectively attack the cancer.

Clinical trials have shown promising results, with some patients experiencing prolonged periods of disease control. However, it's essential to note that not all patients respond equally to immunotherapy, and ongoing research aims to understand the factors influencing treatment outcomes.

Combining immunotherapy with other traditional treatments is also an area of active investigation. The synergy between these modalities could potentially enhance the overall effectiveness of thyroid cancer treatment, providing a more comprehensive approach to managing the disease.

As with any medical advancement, there are challenges and uncertainties. Immunotherapy can have side effects, and identifying biomarkers to predict which patients will benefit the most remains a complex task. Nevertheless, the evolving landscape of immunotherapy for thyroid cancer underscores the continuous effort to improve treatment options and enhance patient outcomes

Emerging Trends in Thyroid Cancer Treatment

In recent years, several emerging trends have shaped the landscape of thyroid cancer treatment, reflecting advancements in research and technology. Here are some notable trends:

1. Immunotherapy Advancements:
   - As mentioned earlier, immunotherapy is gaining attention. Ongoing research explores its potential in thyroid cancer, aiming to enhance the body's immune response against cancer cells.

2. Targeted Therapies:
   - Targeted therapies, which focus on specific molecules involved in cancer growth, are being

investigated. Drugs like tyrosine kinase inhibitors are designed to disrupt signals that promote cancer cell proliferation, offering a more precise and tailored approach.

3. Genomic Profiling:
   - The advent of genomic profiling allows for a better understanding of the genetic alterations driving thyroid cancer. This information can help tailor treatments to specific genetic mutations, potentially improving efficacy.

4. Minimally Invasive Surgical Techniques:
   - Advances in surgical techniques, such as robotic-assisted surgery and endoscopic procedures, are becoming more prevalent. These approaches often result in faster recovery times and reduced postoperative complications.

5. Personalized Medicine:
   - The concept of personalized medicine involves tailoring treatment plans based on individual patient characteristics, including genetics, allowing for more effective and targeted interventions.

6. Multidisciplinary Care:

- A holistic approach to thyroid cancer treatment involves collaboration among various medical specialists, including surgeons, endocrinologists, oncologists, and pathologists. This multidisciplinary approach ensures a comprehensive and well-coordinated strategy.

7. Telemedicine for Follow-up Care:
   - Telemedicine is increasingly being utilized for follow-up care, allowing patients to consult with healthcare providers remotely. This approach can improve accessibility, particularly for those in remote areas or facing mobility challenges.

8. Patient Support and Survivorship Programs:
   - Recognizing the long-term effects of thyroid cancer and its treatment, there's a growing emphasis on survivorship programs. These programs provide support for patients during and after treatment, addressing both physical and emotional aspects of recovery.

9. Advancements in Radioactive Iodine Therapy:
   - Innovations in radioactive iodine therapy aim to optimize its effectiveness while minimizing side effects. Research focuses on refining dosage

regimens and identifying patients who would benefit most from this treatment.

These trends collectively represent a dynamic and evolving landscape in thyroid cancer treatment, with the overarching goal of improving outcomes, minimizing side effects, and enhancing the overall quality of life for individuals affected by this condition.

# Chapter 4

# Lifestyle Approaches for Thyroid Cancer Support

Lifestyle Approaches for Thyroid Cancer Support explores how lifestyle choices can positively influence the well-being of individuals navigating thyroid cancer. From exercise and stress management to sleep hygiene and dietary considerations, this chapter delves into practical strategies that contribute to a holistic and supportive lifestyle. By acknowledging the impact of daily habits on overall health, readers will gain insights into fostering resilience, managing treatment-related challenges, and optimizing their quality of life throughout the thyroid cancer journey. This chapter serves as a guide to empowering individuals to make informed lifestyle choices that complement their medical care and contribute to a sense of well-being.

Nutritional Healing

## - Importance of a Balanced Diet

A balanced diet is crucial for individuals facing thyroid cancer as it plays a pivotal role in overall health and well-being. Adequate nutrition supports the body during cancer treatment, helping to maintain strength, manage treatment-related side effects, and aid in the healing process. For thyroid cancer specifically, ensuring sufficient intake of nutrients like iodine and selenium is essential. A balanced diet also contributes to immune function, energy levels, and overall resilience. Consulting with a healthcare professional or a registered dietitian can help tailor dietary recommendations to individual needs, providing personalized support throughout the thyroid cancer journey.

## - Foods with Anti-Inflammatory Properties

In the context of thyroid cancer, incorporating foods with anti-inflammatory properties into your diet may offer potential benefits. Such foods can help manage inflammation, a factor that can influence overall health. Consider including:

1. Fatty Fish:
   - Rich in omega-3 fatty acids, fish like salmon and mackerel have anti-inflammatory effects, supporting immune function.

2. Berries:
   - Blueberries, strawberries, and raspberries contain antioxidants that may reduce inflammation and contribute to overall well-being.

3. Turmeric:
   - Curcumin, found in turmeric, has potent anti-inflammatory properties. Consider adding turmeric to dishes or trying turmeric supplements.

4. Leafy Greens:
   - Spinach, kale, and other leafy greens are packed with antioxidants and nutrients that can combat inflammation.

5. Nuts and Seeds:
   - Almonds, walnuts, and flaxseeds provide healthy fats and antioxidants, potentially helping to reduce inflammation.

6. Ginger:

- Ginger has anti-inflammatory and antioxidant properties. It can be used in cooking or consumed as ginger tea.

7. Olive Oil:
  - Extra virgin olive oil contains compounds with anti-inflammatory effects. Use it as a primary cooking oil or drizzle it over salads.

8. Green Tea:
  - Rich in polyphenols, green tea has been associated with anti-inflammatory and anticancer effects.

9. Colorful Vegetables:
  - Vegetables like tomatoes, bell peppers, and carrots contain antioxidants that may combat inflammation.

10. Probiotics:
  - Foods like yogurt, kefir, and fermented vegetables can support gut health, influencing inflammation levels.

Incorporating a variety of these foods into a well-balanced diet may contribute to managing inflammation and supporting overall health.

However, it's essential to consult with a healthcare professional or a registered dietitian to ensure dietary choices align with individual health needs and any ongoing treatments.

### - **Nutritional Supplements and Their Role**

Nutritional supplements can play a supportive role in addressing specific nutritional needs during thyroid cancer treatment. However, it's crucial to approach supplementation with guidance from healthcare professionals, as individual requirements vary. Here are some supplements and their potential roles:

1. Iodine:
   - Essential for thyroid function, but supplementation should be approached cautiously, as excess iodine can be detrimental, especially in certain thyroid conditions.

2. Selenium:
   - Some studies suggest selenium's potential in supporting thyroid health. Consultation with a healthcare provider is advised to determine appropriate levels.

3. Vitamin D:
   - Important for bone health and immune function. Deficiency is common, and supplementation may be recommended, especially if sunlight exposure is limited.

4. B Vitamins:
   - Essential for energy metabolism and overall well-being. Adequate intake is vital during cancer treatment.

5. Omega-3 Fatty Acids:
   - Found in fish oil supplements, omega-3s may have anti-inflammatory effects. Consideration of individual health conditions is essential.

6. Calcium:
   - Important for bone health, and supplementation may be advised if dietary intake is insufficient.

7. Protein Supplements:
   - Essential for muscle maintenance, particularly during cancer treatment. Protein shakes or supplements can be beneficial for those with dietary challenges.

8. Antioxidant Supplements:
  - While antioxidants are crucial, obtaining them from whole foods is generally recommended. High-dose antioxidant supplements may interact with treatments, so caution is advised.

Supplementation should be tailored to individual needs, and discussions with healthcare providers are crucial to avoid potential interactions or adverse effects. It's vital to view supplements as complements to a well-balanced diet, emphasizing whole foods whenever possible. Regular monitoring and adjustments, guided by healthcare professionals, ensure a targeted and safe approach to nutritional support during thyroid cancer treatment.

## Physical Activity for Wellness

Let's spotlight the pivotal role of physical activity in enhancing the overall well-being of individuals grappling with thyroid cancer. Beyond conventional treatments, we delve into the profound impact that tailored exercise regimens can have on patients' physical and emotional health. From personalized fitness plans to adaptive exercises, we explore how physical activity not only fosters resilience but may also complement traditional interventions. Join us in uncovering the empowering potential of movement as a catalyst for wellness, as we navigate the nuanced intersection of exercise and thyroid cancer care.

## Exercise and its Impact on Recovery

Amidst the complexities of thyroid cancer recovery, we illuminate the profound and transformative impact of exercise on the physical and emotional well-being of survivors. Beyond its conventional role in fitness, exercise emerges as a therapeutic ally in the journey towards recovery, offering a spectrum of benefits tailored to the unique challenges faced by thyroid cancer patients.

Regular physical activity plays a pivotal role in addressing the physiological aftermath of thyroid cancer treatment. Tailored exercise programs aid in rebuilding strength and stamina, combating the fatigue often associated with treatments such as surgery, radiation, or chemotherapy. Moreover, the cardiovascular benefits of exercise contribute to overall health, potentially offsetting some of the cardiovascular risks associated with certain thyroid cancer therapies.

Beyond the physiological realm, exercise becomes a cornerstone in addressing the psychological and emotional aspects of recovery. The release of endorphins through physical activity not only combats the mental fatigue often experienced post-treatment but also serves as a natural mood enhancer, fostering a positive mindset crucial to the recovery process.

The chapter explores the intricacies of designing personalized fitness regimens, accommodating the unique needs and limitations of thyroid cancer survivors. From low-impact exercises to mindfulness-based movement practices, the narrative unfolds with insights from healthcare professionals and inspiring stories of individuals who have harnessed the healing power of exercise in their thyroid cancer recovery journey.

As we navigate the chapters of recovery, this exploration of exercise as a rejuvenating force underscores its integral role in promoting resilience, restoring vitality, and fostering a renewed sense of well-being for those who have faced the challenges of thyroid cancer.

## Tailored Exercise Plans for Thyroid Cancer Patients

Designing tailored exercise plans for thyroid cancer patients involves a personalized approach that considers their specific health condition, treatment phase, and individual preferences. Here's a step-by-step guide:

1. Assessment:
   - Begin with a comprehensive assessment of the patient's current health status, taking into account the type of thyroid cancer, treatment history, and any associated side effects.
   - Work closely with healthcare professionals, such as oncologists and rehabilitation specialists, to gather relevant information.

2. Communication and Consent:
   - Establish open communication with the patient to understand their preferences, concerns, and any limitations they might be experiencing.

- Obtain consent from the healthcare team and the patient to ensure the exercise plan aligns with their overall treatment goals.

3. Start Slow and Gradual:
   - Begin with low-impact activities like walking, gentle stretching, or tai chi, especially if the patient is in the early stages of recovery.
   - Gradually progress the intensity and duration based on the individual's tolerance and energy levels.

4. Adapt to Treatment Phases:
   - Tailor the exercise plan to accommodate the specific challenges associated with different treatment phases (pre-surgery, post-surgery, radiation, etc.).
   - Modify exercises based on energy levels, potential side effects, and any physical limitations resulting from treatment.

5. Include Strength Training:
   - Integrate light resistance training exercises to rebuild muscle strength, focusing on major muscle groups.
   - Customize the intensity and resistance based on the patient's capabilities.

6. Cardiovascular Exercise:
  - Incorporate cardiovascular exercises like cycling, swimming, or elliptical training to improve overall cardiovascular health.
  - Monitor heart rate and adjust the intensity as needed.

7. Flexibility and Balance:
  - Include gentle stretching exercises to improve flexibility and maintain joint mobility.
  - Incorporate balance exercises to enhance stability, considering any balance issues related to treatment.

8. Mind-Body Connection:
  - Introduce mind-body activities such as yoga or meditation to address stress and support mental well-being.
  - These activities can provide emotional support and relaxation during the recovery process.

9. Regular Monitoring and Adjustments:
  - Regularly assess the patient's progress and modify the exercise plan as needed.

- Encourage ongoing communication to address any changes in the patient's health or treatment status.

10. Individualized Approach:
   - Tailor the exercise plan to the patient's interests and preferences, making it more enjoyable and sustainable.
   - Consider factors like preferred time of day, preferred activities, and any specific likes or dislikes.

Always prioritize safety and consult with healthcare professionals before implementing or modifying an exercise plan for thyroid cancer patients. Individualized guidance from a qualified fitness professional or physical therapist can further enhance the effectiveness and safety of the tailored exercise program.

- **Yoga and its Benefits**

1. Stress Reduction:
   - Visualize yoga as your stress-relief haven, where breathwork and mindful movements ease the burden of dealing with thyroid cancer.

2. Mind-Body Connection:
   - Understand yoga as a conversation between your body and mind, creating a deeper understanding of yourself during the thyroid cancer journey.

3. Gentle Physical Activity:
   - Envision yoga as gentle, tailored movement accessible for all energy levels, addressing the unique needs of thyroid cancer patients.

4. Improved Flexibility and Mobility:
   - Picture yoga contributing to improved flexibility and mobility, particularly addressing challenges post-surgery or related to thyroid symptoms.

5. Energy Restoration:
   - Recognize yoga as a source of energy restoration, countering the fatigue associated with thyroid cancer through mindful movement and breath awareness.

6. Adaptability to Individual Needs:
   - Emphasize the adaptability of yoga to individual preferences and energy levels, allowing a personalized and sustainable approach.

7. Emotional Resilience:
   - Explore how yoga's meditative aspects foster emotional resilience, providing strength and stability in navigating the emotional complexities of thyroid cancer.

8. Community and Support:
   - Introduce the idea of practicing yoga within a supportive community, where shared experiences enhance a sense of support and understanding.

9. Improved Sleep Quality:
   - Highlight the potential benefits of yoga for improving sleep quality, contributing to overall well-being during the thyroid cancer journey.

10. Long-Term Wellness:
   - Conclude by emphasizing yoga as a transformative and ongoing practice, not just exercise, supporting long-term wellness beyond the challenges of thyroid cancer.

   - **Mindfulness Meditation**

1. Introduction to Mindfulness:
   - Imagine diving into the world of mindfulness meditation, a practice that's all about tuning into the

present. See our hero discovering mindfulness as their ally in tackling the stress of dealing with thyroid cancer.

2. Breath Awareness for Calm:
   - Feel the power of breath in mindfulness. Picture scenes where our hero takes a breather, using focused breathing to kick stress and anxiety to the curb.

3. Grounding in the Present Moment:
   - Picture mindfulness as the hero's GPS for the present moment. See them steering clear of worries about the past or future, finding a sense of presence even in the uncertainties of the thyroid cancer journey.

4. Stress Response Regulation:
   - Imagine mindfulness as the hero's superpower, regulating the body's stress response. See them mastering the art of dialing down physiological stress reactions through consistent mindfulness practice.

5. Acceptance and Coping:
   - See mindfulness as the hero's secret weapon for acceptance. Watch as they navigate the emotional

rollercoaster of thyroid cancer with grace, thanks to the equanimity cultivated through mindfulness.

6. Mindful Body Scan for Relaxation
   - Picture the mindful body scan technique in action. Our hero systematically unwinds, bringing attention to different body parts, shedding physical tension linked to stress and illness.

7. Cultivating Emotional Awareness:
   - Picture mindfulness as the hero's emotional radar. Watch them use mindfulness to recognize and process tough emotions tied to their health journey, facing fear, uncertainty, or sadness head-on.

8. Integration into Daily Routine:
   - See mindfulness seamlessly becoming part of our hero's daily routine. It's not just a practice; it's a flexible tool that provides moments of respite wherever they are, easing the demands of thyroid cancer treatment.

9. Mindfulness and Sleep Quality:
   - Explore how mindfulness transforms sleep quality, a crucial element of well-being during the thyroid cancer journey. Picture our hero using

mindfulness techniques for relaxation before bedtime, paving the way for restful nights.

10. Empowerment and Self-Reflection:
    - Conclude by imagining mindfulness as our hero's source of empowerment. See them actively shaping their emotional well-being through self-awareness and resilience. It's not just stress reduction; it's a transformative journey within.

## Deep Breathing Exercises

Deep breathing exercises emerge as a complementary and holistic approach in the treatment of thyroid cancer, offering patients a valuable tool to enhance their overall well-being. Amidst the conventional medical interventions, deep breathing proves instrumental in addressing the physical and emotional dimensions of thyroid cancer.

Physiologically, deep breathing contributes to stress reduction, a crucial aspect in managing the impact of thyroid cancer on both the body and mind. As patients engage in deliberate, slow breaths, the body's stress response is mitigated, leading to a cascade of positive effects. Reduced cortisol levels and enhanced oxygenation promote a more favorable physiological environment for healing.

Furthermore, the practice of deep breathing serves as a vital component in managing symptoms associated with thyroid cancer and its treatments. Patients often experience heightened stress, anxiety, and fatigue, which can be alleviated through the calming effects of intentional breathwork. Improved mental well-being is pivotal in fostering resilience and aiding patients in navigating the emotional complexities of their cancer journey.

Beyond the physiological realm, deep breathing becomes a self-empowering practice for patients. It provides a sense of agency, allowing individuals to actively participate in their healing process. By incorporating deep breathing into their daily routine, patients establish a consistent and accessible means of fostering relaxation, potentially enhancing their overall quality of life.

In conclusion, deep breathing exercises emerge as a valuable adjunctive therapy in the comprehensive treatment of thyroid cancer. By addressing both the physiological and emotional aspects of the disease, deep breathing empowers patients to actively contribute to their well-being, offering a holistic approach that complements conventional medical interventions.

## Stress-Relieving Activities

Stress-relieving activities play a pivotal and comprehensive role in the treatment approach for thyroid cancer patients. Beyond the conventional medical interventions, incorporating stress-relieving activities into the treatment plan acknowledges the intricate interplay between mental and physical health, offering a holistic approach to enhance overall well-being.

One primary benefit of stress-relieving activities in thyroid cancer treatment is their impact on the body's physiological response. Stress, whether derived from the cancer diagnosis, treatment-related challenges, or other life stressors, can exacerbate symptoms and hinder the healing process. Engaging in activities designed to alleviate stress, such as deep breathing exercises, meditation, or yoga, contributes to a reduction in cortisol levels and promotes a more conducive physiological environment for healing.

Moreover, stress-relieving activities serve as a coping mechanism for the emotional challenges associated with thyroid cancer. A cancer diagnosis often induces anxiety, fear, and uncertainty. Incorporating stress-relief practices provides patients with tools to navigate these complex emotions. Techniques like mindfulness meditation offer a space for individuals to acknowledge and accept their feelings, fostering emotional resilience and coping strategies.

The physical symptoms and side effects of thyroid cancer treatment, such as fatigue, pain, or sleep disturbances, can also be ameliorated through stress-relieving activities. Regular engagement in activities like gentle exercise, massage, or aromatherapy can contribute to improved sleep quality, reduced pain perception, and increased energy levels.

Furthermore, stress-relieving activities empower patients by providing a sense of control over their well-being. In the face of a cancer diagnosis, individuals may feel a loss of agency. By actively participating in stress-relieving practices, patients regain a measure of control, fostering a positive mindset and a proactive approach to their treatment journey.

The social aspect of stress-relieving activities should not be overlooked. Participation in support groups, community activities, or group classes tailored for individuals dealing with cancer can create a sense of belonging and understanding. Social connections become integral components of the treatment approach, offering emotional support and a shared experience that alleviates feelings of isolation.

In conclusion, stress-relieving activities form a vital and multidimensional aspect of the treatment approach for thyroid cancer. By addressing physiological, emotional, and social dimensions, these activities contribute to a more comprehensive and patient-centered care strategy, ultimately enhancing the overall quality of life for individuals navigating the complexities of thyroid cancer and its treatment.

- Quality Sleep for Healing

- **Importance of Adequate Sleep**

1. Hormonal Balance: Quality sleep plays a pivotal role in regulating hormones, including those involved in thyroid function. Adequate rest helps maintain a balanced endocrine system, which is essential for managing thyroid cancer.

2. Immune System Support: Sleep is intricately linked to immune function. Getting enough rest strengthens the immune system, aiding the body in its natural defense against cancer cells and supporting the efficacy of medical treatments.

3. Cellular Repair and Growth: During deep sleep, the body engages in cellular repair and growth processes. This is crucial for individuals undergoing thyroid cancer treatment, as it enhances the body's ability to recover from the effects of both the disease and medical interventions.

4. Stress Reduction: Adequate sleep contributes to stress reduction, which is particularly important for thyroid cancer patients. Lower stress levels positively impact overall well-being and may enhance the body's response to treatment.

5. Cognitive Function: Sleep is closely linked to cognitive function and emotional well-being. For individuals facing the challenges of thyroid cancer, maintaining optimal cognitive function through sufficient sleep can improve decision-making and coping abilities.

6. Energy Conservation: Cancer treatments can be physically demanding, leading to fatigue. Quality sleep helps conserve energy, allowing the body to better cope with the side effects of treatments and promoting a faster recovery.

7. Optimizing Medication Efficacy: Sleep can influence the metabolism of medications. Ensuring a proper sleep routine may contribute to the optimal effectiveness of thyroid cancer medications, supporting the overall treatment plan.

8. Psychological Resilience: Coping with a cancer diagnosis involves emotional challenges. Adequate sleep fosters psychological resilience, helping individuals better navigate the emotional aspects of their journey and maintain a positive mindset.

9. Regulating Inflammation: Chronic inflammation is associated with cancer progression. Sleep is known

to have anti-inflammatory effects, potentially aiding in managing inflammation levels during thyroid cancer treatment.

10. Overall Well-being: Good sleep is foundational for overall well-being. It provides a holistic approach to health, supporting not only the physical aspects of treatment but also contributing to mental and emotional strength during the thyroid cancer journey.

## Creating a Relaxing Bedtime Routine

1. Screen-Free Zone: Make your bedroom a screen-free zone at least 30 minutes before bedtime. The blue light emitted by screens can interfere with the production of melatonin, the sleep hormone.

2. Dim the Lights: Lower the lights in your home as bedtime approaches. Dim lighting signals to your body that it's time to wind down and prepares it for sleep.

3. Mindful Breathing: Practice mindful breathing exercises to calm the mind. Deep, slow breaths can

reduce stress and anxiety, creating a conducive environment for a restful night's sleep.

4. Warm Bath or Shower: A warm bath or shower before bedtime can help relax tense muscles and signal to the body that it's time to unwind.

5. Comfortable Sleep Environment: Ensure your bedroom is comfortable and conducive to sleep. Invest in a comfortable mattress and pillows, and keep the room cool and well-ventilated.

6. Aromatherapy: Consider using calming scents like lavender or chamomile. A few drops of essential oil on a pillow or using a diffuser can create a soothing atmosphere.

7. Reading a Relaxing Book: Read a calming or enjoyable book to shift your focus away from daily stressors. Choose something that helps you unwind without stimulating your mind too much.

8. Stretching or Yoga: Gentle stretching or a short yoga session can relax your muscles and alleviate tension, preparing your body for a restful night's sleep.

9. Limit Caffeine and Heavy Meals: Avoid caffeine and heavy meals close to bedtime. Opt for a light snack if needed, and choose decaffeinated beverages in the evening.

10. Establish a Routine: Consistency is key. Establish a regular bedtime routine, going to bed and waking up at the same time each day, even on weekends. This helps regulate your body's internal clock.

11. Journaling: Spend a few minutes jotting down your thoughts in a journal. This can help clear your mind and reduce any lingering stress or worries.

12. Soft Music or White Noise: Play soft, calming music or use a white noise machine to create a soothing auditory environment that promotes relaxation.

Incorporating these elements into your bedtime routine can contribute to a more relaxed and peaceful transition to sleep, improving the overall quality of your rest.

Addressing Sleep Challenges During Treatment

1. Consult with Healthcare Team: Regularly communicate with your healthcare team about any sleep difficulties you are experiencing. They can provide personalized advice based on your specific treatment plan.

2. Establish a Sleep Routine: Create a consistent sleep routine by going to bed and waking up at the same time each day. This helps regulate your body's internal clock, even during treatment.

3. Comfortable Sleep Environment:bEnsure your bedroom is comfortable, cool, and dark. Consider using blackout curtains and adjusting the thermostat to create an optimal sleep environment.

4. Manage Stress: Practice stress-reduction techniques such as meditation, deep breathing, or mindfulness. Managing stress is crucial for promoting better sleep, especially during challenging treatments.

5. Limit Screen Time: Reduce exposure to screens, including smartphones and computers, at least an hour before bedtime. The blue light emitted by

screens can interfere with the production of sleep-inducing hormones.

6. Stay Active: Engage in light, gentle exercise during the day. Physical activity can help improve sleep, but avoid vigorous exercise close to bedtime.

7. Hydration Balance: Be mindful of your hydration, but limit fluid intake close to bedtime to reduce the likelihood of waking up for bathroom trips during the night.

8. Pain Management: If pain is a concern, discuss pain management options with your healthcare provider. Controlling pain can significantly impact your ability to sleep comfortably.

9. Comfortable Bedding: Invest in comfortable bedding, including a supportive mattress and pillows. This can alleviate physical discomfort and enhance your sleep quality.

10. Light Exposure: Get exposure to natural light during the day to help regulate your circadian rhythm. Spend time outdoors or open curtains to let natural light into your living space.

11. Mind-Body Practices: Explore mind-body practices such as guided imagery, progressive muscle relaxation, or gentle yoga to promote relaxation before bedtime.

12. Consult a Sleep Specialist: If sleep challenges persist, consider consulting a sleep specialist. They can conduct a thorough evaluation and provide targeted strategies to address your specific sleep issues during treatment.

Remember that addressing sleep challenges is a dynamic process, and adjustments may be needed based on your evolving health and treatment status. Prioritize open communication with your healthcare team to ensure a comprehensive approach to managing sleep difficulties during treatment.

Hydration and Detoxification

- **Drinking Sufficient Water**

Drinking sufficient water is beneficial for individuals with thyroid cancer in several ways:

1. Medication Absorption: Proper hydration can enhance the absorption of thyroid medications. Staying well-hydrated ensures the effective assimilation of prescribed medications, supporting the management of thyroid cancer.

2. Kidney Function: Hydration is crucial for kidney health, and individuals undergoing thyroid cancer treatment may be exposed to medications that affect kidney function. Adequate water intake supports the kidneys in efficiently processing medications and eliminating waste products.

3. Side Effect Management: Some treatments for thyroid cancer, such as radioactive iodine therapy, may cause side effects like dry mouth and changes in taste. Drinking enough water can help alleviate these symptoms and contribute to overall comfort during treatment.

4. Supporting Immune Function: Hydration is linked to immune function. Proper fluid balance supports the immune system, which is vital for individuals undergoing thyroid cancer treatment to maintain overall health and recovery.

5. Alleviating Fatigue: Treatment for thyroid cancer may lead to fatigue, and staying hydrated is essential for managing energy levels. Dehydration can exacerbate feelings of tiredness, so maintaining adequate fluid intake can contribute to better energy levels.

6. Regulating Body Temperature: Thyroid cancer and its treatment can sometimes affect the body's ability to regulate temperature. Staying hydrated helps support this regulation, especially important during treatments that may impact thermoregulation.

7. Nutrient Transport: Water is a crucial component for transporting nutrients throughout the body. For individuals undergoing treatment, proper hydration aids in nutrient distribution, contributing to overall well-being.

It's important to note that individual hydration needs can vary, and consulting with healthcare professionals is key to understanding specific requirements during thyroid cancer treatment. They can provide personalized advice based on the individual's medical history, treatment plan, and overall health status.

# -Detoxifying Strategies for a Healthy Body

While maintaining a healthy lifestyle is generally beneficial, it's important to note that specific detoxifying strategies are not typically used as primary treatments for thyroid cancer. Treatment for thyroid cancer is primarily medical and may involve surgery, radioactive iodine therapy, hormone therapy, or external beam radiation.

However, adopting a healthy lifestyle can support overall well-being during and after thyroid cancer treatment. Here are some lifestyle strategies that align with a health-focused approach:

1. Nutrient-Rich Diet: Focus on a balanced diet rich in nutrients. Include fruits, vegetables, whole grains, and lean proteins to provide essential vitamins and minerals necessary for overall health and recovery.

2. Hydration: Stay well-hydrated to support the body's natural functions, including kidney health and overall hydration balance.

3. Regular Exercise: Engage in regular physical activity as tolerated, considering your energy levels

and any recommendations from your healthcare team. Exercise can contribute to overall well-being and help manage fatigue.

4. Stress Management: Incorporate stress-reducing practices such as meditation, deep breathing, or yoga. Managing stress is important for overall health and can positively impact the healing process.

5. Adequate Sleep: Prioritize quality sleep to support your body's recovery and natural healing processes.

6. Limit Alcohol and Caffeine: Moderation in alcohol and caffeine consumption can contribute to overall health, considering potential interactions with medications.

7. Consult with Healthcare Professionals: Always consult with your healthcare team before making significant lifestyle changes. They can provide guidance tailored to your individual health status and treatment plan.

It's crucial to approach any health-related strategies in the context of your specific medical condition and treatment plan. Thyroid cancer treatment is best guided by medical professionals who can provide personalized advice based on your individual situation.

- Mind-Body Connection
- **Positive Thinking and Visualization**

Positive thinking and visualization can be beneficial as complementary strategies in managing the emotional and mental aspects of dealing with thyroid cancer. While they aren't substitutes for medical treatments, incorporating these techniques may contribute to overall well-being.

Positive thinking involves cultivating an optimistic outlook, which can positively influence your mental state and potentially impact your body's response to stress. Visualization, on the other hand, entails creating mental images of desired outcomes, promoting a sense of control and reducing anxiety.

When facing thyroid cancer, these techniques might help alleviate stress, improve coping mechanisms, and enhance the overall quality of life. However, it's crucial to maintain open communication with healthcare professionals to ensure a comprehensive and evidence-based approach to treatment.

## - Integrating Holistic Approaches into Treatment

Integrating holistic approaches into the treatment of thyroid cancer involves considering complementary therapies that focus on the overall well-being of the individual, including physical, emotional, and spiritual aspects. Some holistic approaches that may be considered include:

1. Nutrition: Emphasizing a balanced and nutritious diet to support overall health and strengthen the immune system.

2. Mind-Body Techniques: Incorporating stress-reducing practices such as meditation, deep breathing exercises, and yoga to promote relaxation and mental well-being.

3. Acupuncture: Some individuals find acupuncture helpful for managing symptoms like pain and nausea associated with cancer treatments.

4. Herbal Supplements: Discussing with healthcare professionals the potential benefits and risks of herbal supplements that may support conventional treatments.

5. Massage Therapy: Providing comfort and relaxation through gentle massage, which may help manage stress and improve overall mood.

It's crucial to approach holistic therapies as complementary rather than alternative treatments. Always consult with healthcare professionals before incorporating any holistic approaches, ensuring they are safe and compatible with conventional medical treatments for thyroid cancer. Open communication between patients and healthcare providers is key to a comprehensive and well-informed treatment plan.

## - Emotional Well-being and Its Impact on Healing

Emotional well-being plays a significant role in the overall healing process for individuals with thyroid cancer. The mind-body connection is increasingly recognized in medical literature, highlighting the influence of emotional health on physical well-being.

Here are some ways emotional well-being can impact the healing process:

1. Stress Reduction: Managing stress is crucial, as chronic stress may negatively affect the immune system. High stress levels can potentially impact the body's ability to cope with and recover from cancer.

2. Enhanced Immune Function: Positive emotions and a sense of well-being may positively influence the immune system, potentially supporting the body's ability to fight cancer cells and recover from treatments.

3. Adherence to Treatment: Emotional well-being can impact a patient's motivation and adherence to treatment plans. A positive mindset may contribute to better compliance with medical recommendations.

4. Quality of Life: Maintaining emotional well-being can improve the overall quality of life for individuals undergoing thyroid cancer treatment. It may contribute to better coping mechanisms and a more positive outlook.

5. Supportive Relationships: Having a strong support system can positively impact emotional health. Supportive relationships with family, friends, or support groups can provide comfort, encouragement, and understanding during the cancer journey.

While emotional well-being is important, it's essential to recognize that it complements medical treatments rather than serving as a standalone solution. Integrating psychological support, such as counseling or support groups, into the overall treatment plan can be beneficial for addressing emotional aspects and promoting healing in individuals with thyroid cancer.

Social Support and Community Engagement

   **- Building a Support System**

Building a support system is crucial in treating thyroid cancer for several reasons:

1. Emotional Support: Dealing with a cancer diagnosis can be emotionally challenging. A support system, which may include family, friends, or

support groups, provides a crucial emotional anchor. Emotional support can help reduce stress, anxiety, and feelings of isolation.

2. Practical Assistance: Treatment for thyroid cancer may involve medical appointments, procedures, and potential lifestyle adjustments. A support system can offer practical assistance, such as transportation to appointments, help with daily tasks, and emotional understanding during these changes.

3. Information and Advocacy: Having a support system can provide access to information about thyroid cancer, treatment options, and coping strategies. Additionally, individuals in the support network can act as advocates, helping the person navigate the healthcare system and communicate effectively with medical professionals.

4. Motivation and Encouragement: Treatment can be physically demanding, and having a support system provides motivation and encouragement. Positive reinforcement from loved ones can contribute to a more optimistic mindset, which may positively impact the healing process.

5. Reducing Isolation: Cancer diagnosis can lead to feelings of isolation. A support system helps combat this by providing a network of people who care, understand, and are willing to offer companionship and empathy.

6. Enhancing Quality of Life: Building a support system contributes to an improved quality of life during the challenging times of cancer treatment. It helps individuals feel connected, valued, and less burdened by the practical and emotional aspects of the illness.

In summary, a robust support system is a vital component of comprehensive thyroid cancer treatment. It addresses emotional and practical needs, enhances the overall well-being of the individual, and fosters a sense of community during the cancer journey.

- **Participating in Support Groups**

Participating in support groups can be highly beneficial for individuals undergoing thyroid cancer treatment. Here are some advantages:

1. Emotional Support: Support groups offer a safe space to express feelings, fears, and challenges associated with thyroid cancer. Sharing experiences with others who understand can provide comfort and emotional support.

2. Shared Information: Participants in support groups often share valuable information about coping strategies, treatment experiences, and navigating the healthcare system. This shared knowledge can empower individuals with thyroid cancer to make informed decisions about their treatment.

3. Reducing Isolation: Being part of a support group helps combat feelings of isolation that may arise during cancer treatment. Connecting with others who are going through similar experiences fosters a sense of community and understanding.

4. Empowerment: Hearing success stories or learning how others cope with challenges can empower individuals to actively participate in their own treatment and recovery. Support groups can inspire a sense of resilience and hope.

5. Practical Advice: Support groups provide a platform for discussing practical aspects of living with thyroid cancer, such as managing side effects, dietary considerations, and lifestyle adjustments. Practical advice from those who have been through similar experiences can be invaluable.

6. Building Friendships: Long-lasting friendships often form in support groups. These connections extend beyond the shared experience of thyroid cancer, providing ongoing emotional support and camaraderie.

Before joining a support group, individuals should consider factors such as the group's focus, format, and whether it aligns with their preferences. Many organizations, including cancer centers and online platforms, offer diverse support group options, making it easier for individuals to find a group that suits their needs.

### - Engaging with the Thyroid Cancer Community

Engaging with the thyroid cancer community can offer valuable support and resources throughout your journey. Here are ways to connect:

1. Online Forums and Communities: Explore reputable online platforms and forums dedicated to thyroid cancer. Participate in discussions, ask questions, and share your experiences. Websites like CancerConnect, Smart Patients, or Inspire often have active thyroid cancer communities.

2. Social Media Groups: Join thyroid cancer groups on social media platforms like Facebook or Instagram. These groups provide a more interactive and immediate way to connect with individuals facing similar challenges.

3. Attend Support Group Meetings: Many cancer centers or local organizations host regular support group meetings. Attend these sessions to meet others in person, share experiences, and gain insights into coping strategies.

4. Thyroid Cancer Events and Conferences: Attend events or conferences focused on thyroid cancer. These gatherings provide opportunities to connect with experts, learn about the latest research, and meet others in the thyroid cancer community.

5. Collaborate with Advocacy Organizations: Explore involvement with thyroid cancer advocacy

organizations. These groups often provide resources, educational materials, and opportunities to contribute to awareness campaigns or research efforts.

6. Patient Empowerment Programs: Some organizations offer patient empowerment programs specifically tailored to thyroid cancer. These programs may include educational workshops, webinars, and resources to enhance your understanding of the condition and treatment options.

Remember to approach online information with a critical mindset and consult healthcare professionals for personalized advice. Engaging with the thyroid cancer community can provide emotional support, shared experiences, and a sense of empowerment as you navigate your journey.

Holistic Therapies

- **Acupuncture and Acupressure**

Acupuncture and acupressure are complementary therapies originating from traditional Chinese medicine. While they may not treat thyroid cancer directly, some individuals find them beneficial for managing certain symptoms and improving overall well-being during cancer treatment. Here's a brief overview:

1. Acupuncture:
   - What it involves: Thin needles are inserted into specific points on the body to stimulate energy flow (Qi) and promote balance.
   - Potential benefits: Some people report relief from cancer-related symptoms like pain, nausea, and fatigue. It may also help with stress reduction.

2. Acupressure:
   - What it involves: Pressure is applied to specific points on the body using hands, fingers, or devices, instead of needles.
   - Potential benefits: Similar to acupuncture, acupressure may help alleviate symptoms such as nausea, pain, and anxiety. It's non-invasive and can be performed by individuals on themselves.

**For individuals with thyroid cancer:**

- Pain Management: Acupuncture and acupressure may contribute to pain relief, which can be relevant for managing discomfort associated with cancer or its treatments.

- Nausea and Fatigue: Some individuals find these techniques helpful in mitigating nausea and fatigue, common side effects of cancer treatments.

It's crucial to consult with healthcare professionals before incorporating acupuncture or acupressure into your treatment plan. These practices should be viewed as complementary approaches to standard medical care. Inform your healthcare team about any complementary therapies you're considering to ensure they align with your overall treatment and well-being.

## - Massage Therapy

Massage therapy can offer various benefits for individuals undergoing thyroid cancer treatment, although it should be approached with caution and in consultation with healthcare professionals. Here are potential advantages:

1. Stress Reduction: Massage therapy is known for promoting relaxation and reducing stress. Managing

stress is crucial during cancer treatment to support overall well-being.

2. Pain Relief: Gentle massage can help alleviate muscle tension and provide relief from pain, which may be beneficial for individuals experiencing discomfort related to thyroid cancer or its treatments.

3. Improved Sleep Quality: Many cancer patients face challenges with sleep. Massage therapy may contribute to better sleep by promoting relaxation and reducing anxiety.

4. Enhanced Well-Being: The soothing effects of massage can positively impact mental and emotional well-being. It provides a time for individuals to focus on self-care and can contribute to an improved overall mood.

5. Lymphatic Drainage: In some cases, specialized massage techniques, such as lymphatic drainage, may be used to reduce swelling and improve lymphatic circulation, which can be relevant for individuals dealing with lymphedema.

Before incorporating massage therapy into your treatment plan:

- Consultation with Healthcare Team: Discuss your intention to include massage therapy with your healthcare team. They can provide guidance based on your specific medical condition and treatment plan.

- Choose a Certified Practitioner: Ensure that the massage therapist is certified and experienced in working with individuals undergoing cancer treatment. They should be aware of any contraindications or precautions related to your condition.

- Communicate Clearly: Inform the massage therapist about your health condition, treatment details, and any specific concerns or preferences you may have.

Massage therapy can be a valuable component of a holistic approach to cancer care, promoting relaxation and supporting overall well-being.

## - Herbal Remedies and Their Considerations

While herbal remedies are often considered in various health contexts, including cancer, it's crucial to approach them with caution, especially when dealing with a serious condition like thyroid cancer. Here are some considerations:

1. Consult with Healthcare Professionals: Always consult with your healthcare team before using herbal remedies. They can provide guidance based on your specific medical condition, treatment plan, and potential interactions with medications.

2. Potential Interactions: Herbal remedies may interact with medications or other treatments you're undergoing. Some herbs can interfere with the effectiveness of cancer treatments or cause adverse reactions.

3. Safety and Quality: The safety and quality of herbal products can vary. Choose reputable sources and inform your healthcare team about any herbal supplements you're considering.

4. Not a Substitute for Medical Treatment: Herbal remedies should never be used as a substitute for standard medical treatments. They may, at best,

complement conventional therapies and help manage certain symptoms.

5. Commonly Considered Herbs: Some individuals explore herbs like ashwagandha, turmeric, or green tea for their potential anti-inflammatory and antioxidant properties. However, evidence regarding their effectiveness in treating cancer is often preliminary, and more research is needed.

6. Individual Variability: Responses to herbal remedies can vary widely among individuals. What works for one person may not work for another, and there's a lack of standardized dosages for many herbs.

Remember, the field of herbal medicine is still evolving, and research on the effectiveness and safety of specific herbs for cancer treatment is ongoing. Always prioritize evidence-based medical treatments and inform your healthcare team about any complementary therapies you're considering. They can help you make informed decisions that prioritize your health and well-being.

Herbs to use for treating thyroid cancer

While it's essential to approach the topic of using herbs for treating thyroid cancer with caution, as there is limited scientific evidence to support their efficacy as standalone treatments, some herbs have been explored for their potential benefits. It's crucial to emphasize that herbal remedies should not replace conventional medical treatments but may be considered as complementary approaches in consultation with your healthcare team. Here are some herbs that have been studied for their potential impact on thyroid health:

1. Ashwagandha (Withania somnifera):
   - Ashwagandha is an adaptogenic herb that has been traditionally used in Ayurvedic medicine. Some studies suggest that it may have anti-inflammatory and antioxidant properties, which could potentially be beneficial for individuals with thyroid disorders. However, more research is needed to establish its effectiveness and safety in the context of thyroid cancer.

2. Turmeric (Curcuma longa):
   - Curcumin, the active compound in turmeric, is known for its anti-inflammatory and antioxidant

properties. While some studies suggest that turmeric may have potential benefits for managing inflammation and supporting overall health, its direct impact on thyroid cancer specifically is not well-established.

3. Holy Basil (Ocimum sanctum):
   - Holy basil, or tulsi, is another herb with adaptogenic properties. It has been studied for its potential anti-inflammatory and antioxidant effects. While research on its direct impact on thyroid cancer is limited, it may contribute to overall well-being.

4. Guggul (Commiphora wightii):
   - Guggul, derived from the resin of the mukul myrrh tree, has been traditionally used in Ayurvedic medicine. Some studies suggest that guggul may have anti-inflammatory and antioxidant effects, but more research is needed to determine its potential role in thyroid cancer treatment.

5. Siberian Ginseng (Eleutherococcus senticosus):
   - Siberian ginseng is an adaptogenic herb that has been studied for its potential benefits in managing stress and supporting the immune system. Its

impact specifically on thyroid cancer is not well-established.

6. Flaxseed (Linum usitatissimum):
   - Flaxseed is a source of omega-3 fatty acids and lignans, which have been studied for their potential anti-cancer properties. While some research suggests that flaxseed may have benefits for cancer prevention, its role in thyroid cancer specifically is not fully understood.

It's crucial to approach the use of herbs with caution and to consult with your healthcare team before incorporating them into your treatment plan. Some herbs may interact with medications or have contraindications, and their safety and efficacy should be thoroughly discussed with qualified healthcare professionals. Always prioritize evidence-based medical treatments while considering complementary approaches to support overall health during thyroid cancer treatment.

- Environmental Factors


   - Minimizing Exposure to Toxins
Minimizing exposure to toxins is important for overall health, and it can be particularly relevant for

individuals dealing with thyroid cancer or undergoing cancer treatments. Here are some general strategies:

1. Environmental Awareness:
   - Be conscious of environmental pollutants in your surroundings. Limit exposure to industrial chemicals, pesticides, and other potential toxins.
   - Consider using environmentally friendly and non-toxic household products to reduce chemical exposure at home.

2. Healthy Nutrition:
   - Choose organic produce when possible to reduce exposure to pesticides.
   - Be mindful of the quality of seafood, opting for varieties that are low in mercury and other contaminants.

3. Filtered Water:
   - Use a water filter to reduce exposure to contaminants in drinking water. This is especially important if your local water supply may contain pollutants.

4. Limiting Alcohol and Tobacco:

- Minimize or avoid alcohol consumption, as it can contribute to oxidative stress in the body.

- Quit or avoid smoking, as tobacco smoke contains numerous harmful chemicals that can negatively impact health.

5. Safe Food Handling:

- Be cautious with food storage and handling to prevent exposure to foodborne toxins. Follow proper food safety practices.

6. Mindful Personal Care Products:

- Choose personal care products, such as shampoos, lotions, and cosmetics, with fewer chemicals. Look for products labeled as "paraben-free" or "phthalate-free."

7. Air Quality:

- Ensure good ventilation in living spaces to minimize indoor air pollutants.

- Consider using air purifiers if needed, especially if you live in an area with high levels of air pollution.

8. Regular Exercise and Saunas:

- Engage in regular physical activity to support the body's natural detoxification processes.

- Saunas may help eliminate certain toxins through sweating.

9. Consult Healthcare Professionals:
   - Discuss with your healthcare team any concerns about environmental exposures and potential toxins, especially if they may impact your health or cancer treatment.

It's important to note that while these strategies can contribute to overall well-being, they are not a substitute for medical treatment. Always consult with your healthcare professionals for personalized advice based on your specific health condition and treatment plan.

## -Creating a Healthy Living Environment

Creating a healthy living environment is crucial for overall well-being, particularly for individuals dealing with health challenges like thyroid cancer. Here are some tips to promote a healthy living environment:

1. Clean Indoor Air:
   - Ensure good ventilation in your home. Open windows regularly to allow fresh air circulation.

- Use air purifiers to reduce indoor air pollutants, especially if you live in areas with high pollution levels.

2. Non-Toxic Household Products:
- Choose cleaning products, detergents, and other household items that are labeled as non-toxic or environmentally friendly.
- Consider natural alternatives like vinegar and baking soda for cleaning.

3. Reduced Exposure to Allergens:
- Minimize exposure to allergens like dust mites, pet dander, and mold. Regular cleaning and maintenance can help.

4. Safe Drinking Water:
- Use water filters to ensure the quality of your drinking water, especially if there are concerns about contaminants in your local water supply.

5. Healthy Nutrition:
- Opt for organic produce to reduce exposure to pesticides.
- Store food properly to prevent contamination, and maintain a balanced and nutritious diet.

6. Natural Light and Sleep Environment:
   - Maximize exposure to natural light during the day to support circadian rhythms.
   - Create a comfortable and conducive sleep environment by minimizing noise and light at night.

7. Mindful Use of Electronics:
   - Limit screen time before bedtime to promote better sleep.
   - Be mindful of electromagnetic fields (EMFs) by keeping electronic devices at a distance during sleep.

8. Plants Indoors:
   - Indoor plants can help improve air quality by absorbing pollutants and increasing oxygen levels.

9. Safe Personal Care Products:
   - Choose personal care products free from harmful chemicals. Look for products labeled as "paraben-free" or "phthalate-free."

10. Green Spaces and Nature:
   - Spend time in nature or create green spaces within your home, such as potted plants or indoor gardens

11. Reduced Stressors:
   - Create a calm and organized living space to minimize stress. Consider incorporating relaxation techniques like meditation.

12. Safety Measures:
   - Implement safety measures, such as installing smoke detectors and carbon monoxide detectors, to ensure a secure living environment.

Tailor these suggestions to your specific needs and preferences. A healthy living environment can positively impact physical and mental well-being, supporting overall health during thyroid cancer treatment and beyond.

- Personalized Wellness Plans

   - **Collaborating with Healthcare Providers for Personalized Approaches**

Collaborating with healthcare providers is essential for developing personalized approaches to managing thyroid cancer. Here's how you can foster effective collaboration:

1. Open Communication:

- Maintain open and honest communication with your healthcare team. Share your concerns, preferences, and any complementary therapies you are considering

2. Regular Follow-Up Appointments:
   - Attend regular follow-up appointments as scheduled. These appointments allow your healthcare team to monitor your progress, address any issues, and adjust the treatment plan as needed.

3. Ask Questions:
   - Don't hesitate to ask questions about your diagnosis, treatment options, and potential side effects. Understanding your condition empowers you to make informed decisions.

4. Share Your Symptoms:
   - Report any new or changing symptoms promptly. This information helps your healthcare team assess your condition and make necessary adjustments to your treatment plan.

5. Discuss Personalized Goals:

- Work with your healthcare providers to define personalized treatment goals that align with your preferences and priorities.

6. Incorporate Complementary Therapies Safely:
   - If you're considering complementary therapies, discuss them with your healthcare team to ensure they are safe and compatible with your treatment plan.

7. Involve Supportive Care:
   - Integrate supportive care services, such as counseling or support groups, into your overall treatment plan. These services contribute to emotional well-being.

8. Keep a Health Record:
   - Maintain a health record that includes details about your diagnosis, treatments, medications, and any side effects. This record can be valuable during discussions with your healthcare team.

9. Collaborate on Lifestyle Changes:
   - If lifestyle changes are recommended, collaborate with your healthcare team to develop realistic and sustainable plans. This may include

dietary adjustments, exercise, and stress management strategies.

10. Understand Treatment Options:
   - Stay informed about available treatment options, including potential new developments or clinical trials that may be relevant to your case.

Remember, healthcare is a collaborative effort. Your active participation and communication with your healthcare providers contribute to a more personalized and effective approach to managing thyroid cancer.

## - Tailoring Lifestyle Changes to Individual Needs

Tailoring lifestyle changes to individual needs is crucial, especially when managing health conditions like thyroid cancer. Here are key considerations for creating personalized lifestyle adjustments:

1. Consult with Healthcare Professionals:
   - Before making significant lifestyle changes, consult with your healthcare team. They can provide guidance based on your specific health condition, treatment plan, and individual needs.

2. Dietary Modifications:
   - Work with a registered dietitian or nutritionist to tailor dietary changes that meet your nutritional needs. Consider factors such as metabolism, weight management, and potential interactions with medications.

3. Exercise Routine:
   - Customize your exercise routine based on your fitness level, energy levels, and any physical limitations. Aim for a mix of cardiovascular, strength, and flexibility exercises that suit your preferences.

4. Sleep Hygiene:
   - Adapt your sleep routine to your individual needs. Create a comfortable sleep environment, establish a consistent sleep schedule, and address any sleep-related challenges with your healthcare team.

5. Stress Management:
   - Explore stress management techniques that resonate with you. This might include mindfulness, meditation, yoga, or other relaxation methods. Tailor these practices to fit into your daily life.

6. Hydration:
   - Adjust your fluid intake based on your body's needs. Factors like age, climate, and physical activity levels can influence your hydration requirements.

7. Social Support:
   - Consider your social and emotional needs. Build a support system that aligns with your personality and preferences, whether it's through close relationships, support groups, or online communities.

8. Mindfulness and Mental Well-Being:
   - Incorporate mindfulness practices into your routine to support mental well-being. This might include activities like deep breathing exercises, journaling, or spending time in nature.

9. Work-Life Balance:
   - Evaluate your work-life balance and make adjustments as needed. Prioritize self-care and create boundaries to manage stress effectively.

10. Monitor and Adjust:
    - Regularly assess the impact of lifestyle changes on your overall well-being. If necessary, make

adjustments based on your experiences and feedback from your healthcare team.

Remember that individual responses to lifestyle changes can vary, and there is no one-size-fits-all approach. The goal is to create a sustainable and personalized plan that enhances your quality of life while considering the specific challenges and preferences unique to you. Regular communication with healthcare professionals ensures that lifestyle modifications align with your health goals.

# Chapter 5

# Managing Side Effects

Welcome to Chapter 5, where we delve into the crucial aspect of managing side effects during the course of thyroid cancer treatment. This chapter addresses a spectrum of physical and emotional challenges associated with various treatment modalities. From practical strategies for mitigating discomfort to exploring the impact on emotional well-being, we aim to equip you with valuable insights and personalized approaches. Let's navigate the complexities of side effect management, empowering you to foster resilience and maintain a quality life throughout your thyroid cancer journey.

## Coping with Hair Loss

Coping with hair loss, often a side effect of thyroid cancer treatments, can be emotionally challenging. Here are some practical strategies to help navigate this aspect of the cancer journey:

1. Education and Awareness:
   - Understand that hair loss is a common side effect of certain cancer treatments. Knowledge about why it occurs can empower you to cope more effectively.

2. Preparation and Planning:
   - Consider cutting or styling your hair before treatment starts. This can make the transition less abrupt and give you a sense of control.

3. Explore Head Coverings:
   - Experiment with scarves, hats, turbans, or wigs. Find options that make you feel comfortable and confident.

4. Express Yourself:
   - If you choose to wear wigs, explore different styles and colors to express your personal style. Some people find joy in experimenting with new looks.

5. Skin Care:
   - Take care of your scalp by using gentle, fragrance-free products. Moisturize if needed to keep the skin healthy.

6. Share Your Feelings:
   - Talk openly about your feelings with friends, family, or a support group. Sharing your experience can provide emotional relief.

7. Consider Support Groups:
   - Joining a support group for individuals experiencing hair loss due to cancer treatment can provide a sense of community and understanding.

8. Self-Compassion:
   - Be kind to yourself. Understand that it's okay to feel a range of emotions about hair loss. Practice self-compassion and acknowledge your strength in facing this challenge.

9. Focus on Inner Beauty:
   - Remember that true beauty comes from within. Shift your focus to aspects of yourself that are not defined by physical appearance.

10. Maintain a Positive Self-Image:
    - Engage in activities that make you feel good about yourself. Whether it's dressing up, wearing makeup, or pursuing hobbies, maintain a positive self-image.

11. Explore Hair Regrowth Support:
    - If appropriate, explore options for supporting hair regrowth after treatment. Consult with your healthcare team about timelines and potential regrowth strategies.

12. Professional Counseling:
    - Seek professional counseling or therapy if you find that the emotional impact of hair loss is

particularly challenging. A mental health professional can provide guidance and support.

Remember, coping with hair loss is a personal journey, and there is no one-size-fits-all approach. Find what works best for you, and don't hesitate to seek support when needed. You are not alone in facing this aspect of the cancer experience.

## Curbing hair loss

 Hair loss, known as alopecia, is a common side effect of thyroid cancer treatment, particularly due to procedures like thyroidectomy (removal of the thyroid gland) and radiation therapy. While some hair loss may be unavoidable, there are strategies to minimize its impact during thyroid cancer treatment:

1. Nutrient-Rich Diet:
   - Ensure a well-balanced diet with a focus on nutrients vital for hair health. Adequate protein, iron, zinc, and biotin are particularly important. Consult with a nutritionist to tailor your diet to support overall health and hair strength.

2. Gentle Hair Care:

   - Be gentle when washing and brushing your hair. Use a mild shampoo and conditioner, and avoid aggressive brushing or combing to prevent additional stress on weakened hair.

3. Moisturize the Scalp:

   - Keep the scalp moisturized to prevent dryness and irritation. Consider using a mild, hydrating shampoo and conditioner, and avoid harsh chemicals.

4. Avoid Heat Styling:

   - Minimize the use of heat-styling tools like flat irons and blow dryers. Excessive heat can further weaken hair, making it more prone to breakage.

5. Silk or Satin Pillowcase:

   - Use a silk or satin pillowcase, which causes less friction than cotton. This can help reduce hair breakage and minimize stress on the hair.

6. Scalp Massage:

   - Gently massage your scalp to stimulate blood circulation, which may support hair follicles. This can be done using your fingertips in a circular motion.

7. Consider a Shorter Hairstyle:
   - Opt for a shorter hairstyle, as shorter hair may appear fuller and be less noticeable during periods of hair loss.

8. Protect Hair from the Sun:
   - When outdoors, protect your head and hair from the sun using hats or scarves. This helps shield your hair from potential damage due to sun exposure.

9. Wig or Head Coverings:
   - Consider using wigs, scarves, or other head coverings if hair loss becomes more extensive. This can provide a sense of normalcy and boost confidence.

10. Mind-Body Techniques:
    - Engage in stress-relieving activities like meditation, yoga, or deep breathing. While not a direct prevention method, managing stress can positively impact overall health and well-being, potentially influencing hair health.

11. Stay Hydrated:

- Proper hydration is essential for overall health, including hair health. Drink enough water to maintain hydration.

12. Consult with a Dermatologist:*
   - Seek advice from a dermatologist who specializes in hair and scalp health. They can provide personalized recommendations and treatments to support your hair during and after thyroid cancer treatment.

It's crucial to note that individual responses to treatment and the extent of hair loss can vary. Discuss your concerns and preferences with your healthcare team, as they can provide guidance tailored to your specific situation.

- Dealing with Fatigue

   Dealing with fatigue, a common side effect of thyroid cancer and its treatments, requires a holistic approach. Here are practical strategies to manage and cope with fatigue:

1. Prioritize Rest:

- Listen to your body and rest when needed. Allow yourself breaks throughout the day, and ensure you are getting adequate sleep at night.

2. Maintain a Regular Sleep Schedule:
   - Establish a consistent sleep routine. Aim for a set bedtime and wake-up time to support better sleep quality.

3. Stay Hydrated:
   - Dehydration can contribute to fatigue. Drink plenty of water throughout the day to stay hydrated.

4. Balanced Nutrition:
   - Consume a well-balanced diet rich in nutrients. Consider consulting with a nutritionist to ensure you are getting the necessary fuel for your body.

5. Manage Stress:
   - Practice stress management techniques, such as meditation, deep breathing exercises, or yoga. Chronic stress can exacerbate fatigue.

6. Light Exercise:
   - Engage in light, gentle exercise such as walking or stretching. Regular physical activity can improve energy levels.

7. Pacing Activities:
 - Break tasks into smaller, manageable steps and pace yourself throughout the day to conserve energy.

8. Ask for Help:
 - Don't hesitate to delegate tasks or ask for help when needed. Friends and family may be willing to assist with daily responsibilities.

9. Mindful Caffeine Use:
 - Use caffeine judiciously. While it can provide a temporary energy boost, excessive caffeine intake may disrupt sleep patterns.

10. Set Realistic Goals:
 - Establish achievable goals and prioritize tasks. Understand that it's okay to adjust expectations during periods of fatigue.

11. Socialize and Seek Support:
 - Maintain social connections and seek support from friends, family, or support groups. Sharing your feelings and experiences can provide emotional relief.

12. Address Underlying Causes:
   - Work with your healthcare team to identify and address any underlying medical factors contributing to fatigue.

13. Professional Support:
   - If fatigue persists or becomes overwhelming, consult with healthcare professionals or specialists who can provide guidance on managing and addressing persistent fatigue.

Remember that managing fatigue is an ongoing process, and it's essential to communicate openly with your healthcare team. Tailor these strategies to your individual needs, and be patient with yourself as you navigate the challenges associated with fatigue during thyroid cancer treatment.

- Emotional Well-being

Maintaining emotional well-being during thyroid cancer treatment is essential for overall quality of life. Here are strategies to support emotional well-being:

1. Open Communication:

- Communicate openly with your healthcare team, friends, and family about your emotions, concerns, and needs.

2. Support System:
   - Cultivate a strong support system. Surround yourself with people who understand and provide encouragement.

3. Mindfulness and Relaxation:
   - Practice mindfulness and relaxation techniques, such as deep breathing, meditation, or yoga, to manage stress and promote emotional balance.

4. Counseling or Therapy:
   - Consider professional counseling or therapy to address emotional challenges and develop coping strategies.

5. Express Yourself:
   - Express your feelings through writing, art, or talking. Creative outlets can be therapeutic.

6. Set Realistic Expectations:
   - Manage expectations and set realistic goals. Be kind to yourself and recognize the value of small achievements.

7. Engage in Activities You Enjoy:
   - Continue or discover activities that bring joy and fulfillment. Engaging in hobbies and interests can uplift your spirits.

8. Stay Connected:
   - Maintain social connections. Even if it's through virtual means, staying connected with others is vital for emotional well-being.

9. Educate Yourself:
   - Learn about thyroid cancer, treatments, and potential side effects. Knowledge can empower and reduce uncertainty.

10. Positive Affirmations:
   - Incorporate positive affirmations into your daily routine. Affirmations can foster a positive mindset.

11. Gratitude Practice:
   - Cultivate a gratitude practice by reflecting on aspects of your life for which you are thankful. This can shift focus towards the positive.

12. Monitor Mental Health:

- Keep track of your mental health and seek professional help if you notice persistent feelings of sadness, anxiety, or depression.

13. Engage in Support Groups:
- Participate in support groups or forums where you can connect with others facing similar challenges. Sharing experiences can provide comfort and understanding.

Remember that emotional well-being is a dynamic process, and it's okay to seek help when needed. Prioritize self-care, and acknowledge the importance of your emotional health as an integral part of your overall well-being during thyroid cancer treatment.

# Chapter 6

# Survivorship and Follow-up Care

## Life After Treatment

Life after thyroid cancer treatment marks a significant transition, and it comes with both relief and adjustments. Here are key considerations for navigating the post-treatment phase:

1. Follow-Up Care:
   - Attend regular follow-up appointments with your healthcare team to monitor your health and address any concerns. Regular check-ups are crucial for long-term well-being.

2. Emotional Well-Being:
   - Continue prioritizing your emotional well-being. If needed, seek ongoing support from counselors, support groups, or mental health professionals.

3. Healthy Lifestyle:

- Maintain a healthy lifestyle with a balanced diet, regular exercise, and adequate sleep. These habits contribute to overall well-being and may help prevent recurrence.

4. Thyroid Hormone Replacement Therapy:
   - If you underwent thyroid surgery, continue with any prescribed thyroid hormone replacement therapy. Regular monitoring ensures optimal hormone levels.

5. Body Image and Self-Esteem:
   - Address any changes in body image or self-esteem that may have occurred during treatment. Seek support or counseling if necessary.

6. Fatigue and Energy Levels:
   - Gradually reintroduce physical activity into your routine. Listen to your body and pace yourself to manage any lingering fatigue.

7. Communication with Healthcare Team:
   - Maintain open communication with your healthcare team about any new symptoms, concerns, or changes in your health.

8. Screening for Recurrence:

- Understand the importance of ongoing surveillance and screening for potential recurrence. Work with your healthcare team to establish a plan for long-term monitoring.

9. Financial and Career Considerations:
   - Address any financial or career concerns that may have arisen during treatment. This may involve discussing work accommodations or seeking financial guidance.

10. Family and Relationships:
    - Nurture relationships with family and friends. Share your experiences and feelings, and seek support if needed.

11. Future Planning:
    - Consider your long-term goals and aspirations. Life after treatment is an opportunity to reassess priorities and make plans for the future.

12. Celebrate Milestones:
    - Acknowledge and celebrate milestones in your recovery. Reflect on the progress you've made and the resilience you've shown.

13. Cancer Survivorship Programs:
   - Explore cancer survivorship programs offered by healthcare institutions. These programs often provide resources and support tailored to individuals post-treatment.

Remember that the post-treatment phase is unique for each person, and adjustments may take time. Regular communication with your healthcare team, a focus on holistic well-being, and a positive mindset can contribute to a fulfilling and healthy life after thyroid cancer treatment.


   - Regular Check-ups and Monitoring

Regular check-ups and monitoring are essential components of post-treatment care for thyroid cancer. Here's why they are important and what to expect:

1. Detecting Recurrence:
   - Regular check-ups enable healthcare professionals to monitor for any signs of thyroid cancer recurrence. Early detection is crucial for effective management.

2. Thyroid Hormone Levels:
   - Monitoring thyroid hormone levels is especially relevant if you underwent thyroid surgery. Adjustments to hormone replacement therapy can be made as needed to maintain optimal levels.

3. Imaging Studies:
   - Periodic imaging studies, such as neck ultrasound or other scans, may be conducted to assess the status of the thyroid bed and surrounding tissues.

4. Blood Tests:
   - Blood tests, including thyroid function tests and tumor marker tests, may be part of routine monitoring to evaluate overall health and the potential presence of cancer.

5. Physical Examinations:
   - Regular physical examinations, including palpation of the neck, help healthcare professionals assess for any changes or abnormalities.

6. Discussion of Symptoms:
   - During check-ups, discuss any new symptoms or concerns you may be experiencing. Open communication helps address issues promptly.

7. Psychosocial Support:
   - Beyond physical monitoring, check-ups offer an opportunity to discuss psychosocial aspects of survivorship, including emotional well-being and any challenges you may be facing.

8. Lifestyle and Well-being:
   - Healthcare professionals may inquire about your lifestyle, diet, exercise, and overall well-being. Addressing these aspects contributes to your long-term health.

9. Education and Guidance:
   - Check-ups provide an opportunity for ongoing education and guidance. Stay informed about self-care practices and potential signs to watch for between appointments.

10. Individualized Care Plans:
   - Your healthcare team will tailor a care plan based on your specific situation and any potential risk factors. This individualized approach ensures that your post-treatment care aligns with your needs.

11. Long-Term Survivorship:

- Regular monitoring is part of long-term survivorship care, emphasizing not only cancer detection but also overall health promotion and preventive measures.

12. Cancer Survivorship Programs:
   - Explore cancer survivorship programs offered by healthcare institutions. These programs often provide resources, support, and guidance for individuals post-treatment.

13. Advocacy for Yourself:
   - Take an active role in your care. Advocate for yourself by discussing any concerns, asking questions, and actively participating in the decision-making process.

Regular check-ups and monitoring create a comprehensive framework for post-treatment care, emphasizing early detection, health maintenance, and ongoing support. Collaborate closely with your healthcare team to ensure that your post-treatment plan is tailored to your individual needs and promotes a healthy and fulfilling life after thyroid cancer.

# Chapter 7

# Prevention and Early Detection Strategies

In this pivotal chapter, we explore proactive measures for preventing and detecting thyroid cancer early. From lifestyle considerations to screening techniques, we delve into strategies that empower individuals

## Thyroid Health Practices

Maintaining thyroid health involves adopting practices that support its proper functioning. Consider the following strategies for promoting thyroid well-being:

1. Iodine-Rich Diet:
   - Consume iodine-rich foods, such as seafood, dairy products, and iodized salt, to support thyroid hormone production. However, avoid excessive iodine intake.

2. Balanced Nutrition:

- Maintain a balanced diet with essential nutrients like selenium, zinc, and vitamin D, which play roles in thyroid function. Consult with a healthcare professional or dietitian for personalized advice.

3. Limit Soy Intake:

- If you have thyroid concerns, moderate your intake of soy products as they may interfere with thyroid hormone absorption.

4. Regular Exercise:

- Engage in regular physical activity to support overall health and metabolism. Exercise contributes to hormonal balance and can aid in weight management.

5. Adequate Sleep:

- Prioritize sufficient and quality sleep. Sleep is essential for hormone regulation, including those produced by the thyroid.

6. Stress Management:

- Practice stress reduction techniques such as meditation, deep breathing, or yoga. Chronic stress can impact thyroid function.

7. Regular Check-ups:
   - Schedule regular check-ups with a healthcare professional to monitor thyroid health. Discuss any symptoms or concerns promptly.

8. Limit Environmental Toxins:
   - Be mindful of exposure to environmental toxins. Minimize contact with pollutants and chemicals that can potentially affect thyroid function.

9. Limit Goitrogenic Foods:
   - Goitrogens are substances that may interfere with thyroid function. While some are healthy, consider moderation in consumption of raw cruciferous vegetables like broccoli and cabbage.

10. Avoid Excessive Supplements:
   - Avoid excessive intake of iodine or other thyroid-related supplements without medical guidance. Balance is key to maintaining thyroid health.

11. Know Your Family History:
   - Be aware of your family's medical history, as thyroid conditions can have a genetic component. Inform your healthcare provider of any family history of thyroid issues.

12. Thyroid Health Screenings:
  - If you have a family history or other risk factors, discuss thyroid health screenings with your healthcare provider. Early detection is crucial for effective management.

Remember, individual health needs may vary, and these practices should be tailored to your specific situation. Consult with healthcare professionals for personalized advice and guidance on maintaining optimal thyroid health.

## Importance of Regular Health Check-ups

Regular health check-ups play a crucial role in maintaining overall well-being and preventing potential health issues. Here are key reasons highlighting the importance of regular check-ups:

1. Early Detection of Health Issues:
  - Regular check-ups facilitate the early detection of health problems, allowing for prompt intervention and improved treatment outcomes.

2. Preventive Care:
   - Health check-ups include preventive measures such as vaccinations, screenings, and lifestyle advice to reduce the risk of developing certain conditions.

3. Monitoring Chronic Conditions:
   - For individuals with chronic conditions, regular check-ups help monitor the condition's progression, adjust treatment plans, and manage symptoms effectively.

4. Health Maintenance:
   - Routine check-ups contribute to maintaining good health by addressing potential risk factors, providing nutritional advice, and promoting healthy lifestyle choices.

5. Blood Pressure and Cholesterol Management:
   - Regular monitoring of blood pressure and cholesterol levels helps identify and manage cardiovascular risk factors, reducing the likelihood of heart-related issues

6. Cancer Prevention and Early Detection:
   - Health screenings and examinations are vital for detecting cancers early when treatment is often

more successful. Regular check-ups include screenings based on age, gender, and risk factors.

7. Mental Health Support:
  - Regular check-ups offer opportunities to discuss mental health concerns. Healthcare providers can provide guidance, referrals, or interventions to support emotional well-being.

8. Thyroid Health and Hormone Levels:
  - For individuals with thyroid concerns or hormonal imbalances, regular check-ups allow for monitoring thyroid function and adjusting hormone levels as needed.

9. Health Education:
  - Check-ups provide opportunities for healthcare professionals to educate individuals on health-related topics, including nutrition, exercise, and disease prevention.

10. Immunizations:
  - Routine check-ups ensure that individuals are up-to-date on vaccinations, protecting against preventable diseases and contributing to community immunity.

11. Eye and Dental Health:
   - Regular check-ups extend to eye and dental health, addressing issues early and preventing complications.

12. Healthy Aging:
   - As individuals age, regular check-ups become increasingly important for managing age-related health concerns and maintaining a good quality of life.

13. Establishing a Relationship with Healthcare Providers:
   - Regular visits help establish a relationship with healthcare providers, fostering open communication and trust. This relationship is valuable for personalized care and prompt attention to health needs.

Prioritizing regular health check-ups is a proactive approach to well-being, enabling individuals to take control of their health, identify potential issues early, and work collaboratively with healthcare professionals to maintain a healthy and fulfilling life.

## Coping Strategies for Patients and Caregivers

Coping with a health challenge like thyroid cancer involves both patients and caregivers. Here are coping strategies for both:

**For Patients:**

1. Open Communication:
   - Communicate openly with your healthcare team, expressing concerns and seeking clarification about your condition and treatment.

2. Build a Support System:
   - Cultivate a strong support system with family, friends, and support groups. Sharing your experiences and feelings can provide emotional relief.

3. Self-Care Practices:
   - Prioritize self-care, including adequate sleep, nutrition, and exercise. Taking care of your overall well-being supports resilience during treatment.

4. Set Realistic Goals:

- Establish achievable short-term and long-term goals. Celebrate small victories and progress in your recovery.

5. Mindfulness and Stress Reduction:
   - Practice mindfulness techniques, such as meditation or deep breathing, to manage stress and promote emotional balance.

6. Educate Yourself:
   - Learn about thyroid cancer, treatment options, and potential side effects. Knowledge empowers you to make informed decisions and actively participate in your care.

7. Express Your Feelings:
   - Articulate your emotions through writing, art, or conversations. Expressing your feelings can be therapeutic.

8. Engage in Activities You Enjoy:
   - Continue engaging in activities that bring you joy and fulfillment. Pursuing hobbies and interests can provide a sense of normalcy.

9. Professional Support:

- Consider seeking professional counseling or therapy to address emotional challenges. A mental health professional can provide guidance and support.

**For Caregivers**:

1. Communication and Understanding:
   - Maintain open communication with the patient. Understand their feelings, concerns, and preferences regarding treatment and support.

2. Self-Care:
   - Attend to your own well-being. Take breaks, prioritize sleep, and engage in activities that recharge you. Caring for yourself enables you to better support the patient.

3. Educate Yourself:
   - Learn about thyroid cancer, treatment processes, and potential challenges. Being informed helps you provide more effective support.

4. Seek Support for Yourself:
   - Connect with other caregivers, either through support groups or online communities. Sharing

experiences with others in similar roles can be comforting.

5. Encourage Open Communication:
   - Encourage the patient to express their feelings and concerns. Create a supportive environment where they feel heard and understood.

6. Be Flexible and Adaptable:
   - Recognize that the caregiving journey may involve unexpected changes. Be flexible and adaptable to the evolving needs of the patient.

7. Coordinate with Healthcare Team:
   - Collaborate with the healthcare team to stay informed about the patient's treatment plan and any adjustments needed. Your involvement is valuable.

8. Offer Practical Assistance:
   - Provide practical assistance with daily tasks, transportation to appointments, and coordinating with healthcare providers. This support can alleviate the patient's burden.

Remember, both patients and caregivers benefit from open communication, mutual understanding, and a collaborative approach to managing the challenges of thyroid cancer. Seeking support when needed and maintaining a balanced approach to well-being contribute to a more resilient journey for both individuals involved.

# Conclusion

Recap of Key Takeaways

1. Thyroid Cancer Treatment Approach:
   - Treatment often involves a combination of surgery, radioactive iodine therapy, and hormone replacement therapy.

2. Holistic Approaches:
   - Integrating holistic approaches, including positive thinking, visualization, and lifestyle changes, can complement medical treatment for thyroid cancer.

3. Emotional Well-being:
   - Emotional well-being significantly impacts healing. Coping strategies, support systems, and professional assistance play crucial roles in managing the emotional aspects of thyroid cancer.

4. Support System Importance
   - Building and maintaining a strong support system is essential in navigating the challenges of thyroid cancer. Support groups and community engagement provide valuable resources.

5. Complementary Therapies:

  - Complementary therapies like acupuncture, acupressure, massage therapy, and herbal remedies may contribute to overall well-being. Always consult with healthcare providers before incorporating these into your regimen.

6. Minimizing Toxins and Creating Healthy Environments:

  - Minimizing exposure to toxins and creating a healthy living environment is crucial for individuals dealing with thyroid cancer. Consider factors like air quality, household products, and personal care items.

7. Collaboration with Healthcare Providers:

  - Collaborating with healthcare providers is key. Maintain open communication, attend regular follow-ups, and actively engage in discussions about treatment options and goals.

8. Tailoring Lifestyle Changes:

  - Tailor lifestyle changes to individual needs. Consider diet modifications, exercise routines, stress management, and sleep hygiene based on personal preferences and health status.

9. Managing Side Effects:
   - Chapter 6 focuses on managing side effects, encompassing physical and emotional well-being. Strategies include open communication, personalizing coping mechanisms, and engaging in support systems.

10. Life After Treatment:
    - Life after thyroid cancer treatment involves regular follow-up care, emotional well-being prioritization, and considerations for overall health and future planning.

11. Prevention and Early Detection:
    - Chapter 8 explores prevention and early detection strategies, emphasizing lifestyle choices, screenings, and proactive healthcare practices.

12. Thyroid Health Practices:
    - Maintain thyroid health through practices like a balanced diet, exercise, stress management, and avoiding excessive exposure to environmental factors.

13. Regular Health Check-ups:

- Regular health check-ups are crucial for early detection of health issues, preventive care, and monitoring chronic conditions. They contribute to overall well-being and a proactive approach to health.

14. Coping Strategies for Patients and Caregivers:
- Patients benefit from open communication, self-care practices, and seeking professional support. Caregivers should prioritize their own well-being, educate themselves, and offer practical assistance while fostering open communication.

Remember, each individual's journey with thyroid cancer is unique, and these takeaways provide a comprehensive overview to guide and empower individuals on this path. Always consult with healthcare professionals for personalized advice and support.

Empowering Readers for a Healthier Future

Empowering readers for a healthier future involves providing knowledge, fostering a proactive mindset, and encouraging positive lifestyle choices. Here are key strategies for achieving this empowerment:

1. Knowledge and Education:
   - Equip readers with comprehensive and accurate information about thyroid health, cancer, and treatment options. Knowledge is a powerful tool for making informed decisions.

2. Proactive Health Management:
   - Encourage a proactive approach to health by emphasizing preventive measures, regular health check-ups, and early detection practices. Empower readers to take an active role in their well-being.

3. Holistic Well-being:
   - Highlight the importance of holistic well-being, encompassing physical, emotional, and mental health. Advocate for lifestyle choices that promote overall wellness.

4. Individualized Strategies:
   - Recognize the uniqueness of each individual's health journey. Encourage readers to tailor lifestyle changes, coping strategies, and treatment decisions to their specific needs and preferences.

5. Building Support Systems:

- Emphasize the significance of building and maintaining strong support systems. Support from friends, family, and healthcare professionals plays a crucial role in facing health challenges.

6. Navigating Challenges with Resilience:
   - Foster resilience by addressing challenges openly, providing coping mechanisms, and highlighting the importance of adaptability in the face of health-related uncertainties.

7. Community Engagement:
   - Promote community engagement through support groups, online forums, and participation in health-focused communities. Sharing experiences and insights creates a sense of connection and understanding.

8. Encouraging Healthy Practices:
   - Encourage healthy practices, including balanced nutrition, regular exercise, stress management, and sufficient sleep. These habits contribute to long-term well-being.

9. Advocacy for Personalized Care:
   - Advocate for personalized and patient-centered care. Empower readers to actively communicate

with healthcare providers, ask questions, and actively participate in decision-making.

10. Positive Mindset and Future Planning:
   - Cultivate a positive mindset by focusing on achievements, setting realistic goals, and envisioning a healthier future. Encourage readers to plan for their future health and well-being.

11. Continued Learning:
   - Promote a culture of continued learning about health and wellness. Encourage readers to stay informed, ask questions, and seek updated information on thyroid health and related topics.

12. Celebrating Victories:
   - Celebrate personal victories, whether small or significant, on the health journey. Recognizing achievements fosters motivation and a positive outlook.

Empowering readers for a healthier future involves a collaborative effort between healthcare providers, individuals, and communities. By providing comprehensive information, fostering a proactive mindset, and encouraging healthy practices, readers can embark on a journey toward a future characterized by informed decisions, resilience, and overall well-being.

Made in the USA
Las Vegas, NV
20 December 2023

83378523R00085